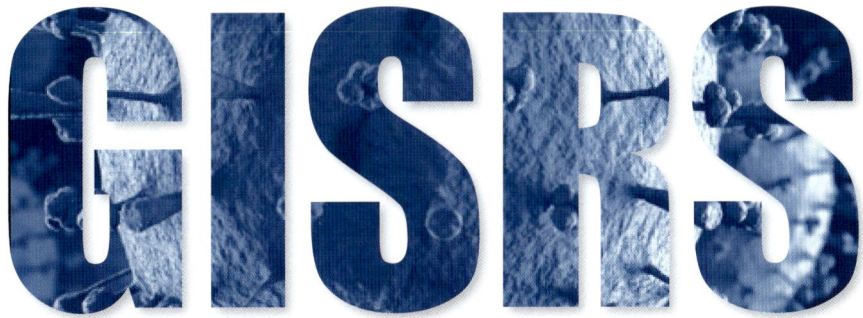

GISRS
Global Influenza Surveillance and Response System

Uniting the world in the fight against influenza

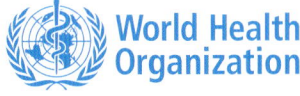

Uniting the world in the fight against influenza: the global influenza surveillance and response system

ISBN 978-92-4-156562-2

© **World Health Organization 2018**

Some rights reserved. This work is available under the Creative Commons Attribution-NonCommercial-ShareAlike 3.0 IGO licence (CC BY-NC-SA 3.0 IGO; https://creativecommons.org/licenses/by-nc-sa/3.0/igo).

Under the terms of this licence, you may copy, redistribute and adapt the work for non-commercial purposes, provided the work is appropriately cited, as indicated below. In any use of this work, there should be no suggestion that WHO endorses any specific organization, products or services. The use of the WHO logo is not permitted. If you adapt the work, then you must license your work under the same or equivalent Creative Commons licence. If you create a translation of this work, you should add the following disclaimer along with the suggested citation: "This translation was not created by the World Health Organization (WHO). WHO is not responsible for the content or accuracy of this translation. The original English edition shall be the binding and authentic edition".

Any mediation relating to disputes arising under the licence shall be conducted in accordance with the mediation rules of the World Intellectual Property Organization.

Suggested citation. Uniting the world in the fight against influenza: the global influenza surveillance and response system. Geneva: World Health Organization; 2018. Licence: CC BY-NC-SA 3.0 IGO.

Cataloguing-in-Publication (CIP) data. CIP data are available at http://apps.who.int/iris.

Sales, rights and licensing. To purchase WHO publications, see http://apps.who.int/bookorders.
To submit requests for commercial use and queries on rights and licensing, see http://www.who.int/about/licensing.

Third-party materials. If you wish to reuse material from this work that is attributed to a third party, such as tables, figures or images, it is your responsibility to determine whether permission is needed for that reuse and to obtain permission from the copyright holder. The risk of claims resulting from infringement of any third-party-owned component in the work rests solely with the user.

General disclaimers. The designations employed and the presentation of the material in this publication do not imply the expression of any opinion whatsoever on the part of WHO concerning the legal status of any country, territory, city or area or of its authorities, or concerning the delimitation of its frontiers or boundaries. Dotted and dashed lines on maps represent approximate border lines for which there may not yet be full agreement.

The mention of specific companies or of certain manufacturers' products does not imply that they are endorsed or recommended by WHO in preference to others of a similar nature that are not mentioned. Errors and omissions excepted, the names of proprietary products are distinguished by initial capital letters.

All reasonable precautions have been taken by WHO to verify the information contained in this publication. However, the published material is being distributed without warranty of any kind, either expressed or implied. The responsibility for the interpretation and use of the material lies with the reader. In no event shall WHO be liable for damages arising from its use.

Design and layout by Morfa Inc., Ottawa, Canada

Printed in France

Contents

Foreword — v

Acknowledgements — vi

Preface — vii

1   Influenza – a global threat requiring a global response — 1

2   1918–1947 – aftermath of a devastating pandemic — 11

3   1947–1952 – the birth of GISRS — 19

4   GISRS – a public health resource for the world — 25

5   From WHO recommendations to seasonal influenza vaccine production — 35

6   Preparing for the next pandemic – constant vigilance and readiness to respond — 43

7   A long history of responding to emergencies — 53

8   Harnessing technology and furthering knowledge — 63

9   Working together – the driving force of GISRS — 71

10   Looking to the future — 81

The GISRS Journey — 88

Foreword

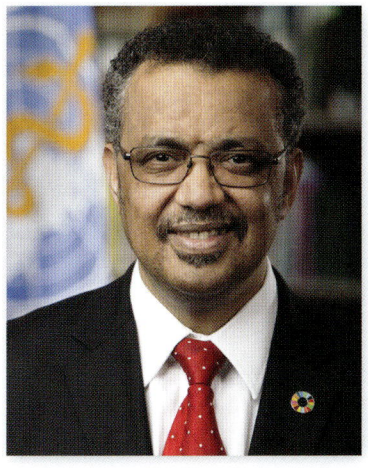

For centuries, influenza viruses have presented a formidable and ever-evolving threat to humankind, causing untold individual suffering and wreaking economic havoc on communities worldwide. Latest estimates indicate that up to 650 000 deaths occur each year as the direct result of seasonal influenza – a significant increase on previous estimates and a stark indication of the recurring social and economic burden caused by such epidemics.

Furthermore, when faced with the threat of an influenza pandemic, history and growing scientific awareness have taught us that we must be able to act quickly and decisively. The 1918 Spanish flu pandemic remains one of the worst global health disasters ever to befall the human race, with an estimated 3% of the world's entire population perishing in a matter of months. In today's increasingly interconnected world, deadly infectious diseases can affect anyone, anywhere. That's why global health security is one of three strategic priorities in the Thirteenth General Programme of Work of the World Health Organization (WHO), with a target to see 1 billion people better protected from health emergencies by 2023. Maintaining a globally coordinated network dedicated to protecting the world from influenza in all its forms is a vital part of achieving that goal.

I am proud to say that WHO, through its Global Influenza Programme, has been at the very heart of the Global Influenza Surveillance and Response System (GISRS) since its creation in 1952. Now in its seventh decade, GISRS continues to be a truly global mechanism for international collaboration in monitoring and responding to influenza viruses, as well as other dangerous respiratory viruses. Over the course of its existence, generations of scientists in countries worldwide have worked together through GISRS to make the world a safer place.

In 2017, GISRS reached its landmark 65th year – for many individuals the milestone for retirement. But we live in a world still facing the recurring and very real threat of influenza and so the mission of GISRS remains far from accomplished. Instead, this global public health resource remains vital, with its ever-increasing global reach and continuing determination to drive and harness new and exciting technological advances. I warmly welcome the opportunity provided by this book not only to look back and celebrate 65 years of this unique and enduring example of international health collaboration at its finest, but also to look forward as GISRS meets the challenges of the next 65 years.

Dr Tedros Adhanom Ghebreyesus
DIRECTOR-GENERAL, WORLD HEALTH ORGANIZATION

Acknowledgements

The WHO Global Influenza Programme would like to acknowledge the contributions made by current and retired GISRS colleagues to the development of this book. The photographs and other documents provided by them have been invaluable. Thanks are extended to staff in the WHO Archives, WHO Library and WHO Press for their professional guidance and help. Acknowledgement is also made of the support for this project provided by the WHO Office of the Director-General, and the WHO Office of the Deputy Director-General of Emergency Preparedness and Response (and formerly by the WHO Office of the Assistant Director-General of Health, Security and the Environment). Special thanks are also due to the WHO Collaborating Centre for Reference and Research on Influenza within the Centers for Disease Control and Prevention, Atlanta, Georgia, United States of America (USA) for its generous financial support for the development of this book.

Research / Historical Work	Reynald Erard and Marie Villemin Partow (WHO Archives), Maja Lièvre, Lukas Schemper, Thedi Ziegler
Content Developers	Tony Waddell, Thedi Ziegler
Designer	Derek Ellis
Reviewers	Nancy Cox, Alan Hay, Ann Moen, John Wood, Thedi Ziegler
Core Group	Derek Ellis, Awandha Mamahit, Tony Waddell, Wenqing Zhang

Preface

GISRS is a truly unique global public health achievement and one of the most enduring international public health collaborations in history. From its early beginnings as a network of 26 laboratories, GISRS now encompasses more than 150 laboratories in more than 100 countries. These laboratories provide the expertise needed to vigilantly monitor and quickly respond to the continuous threat posed by seasonal, zoonotic and pandemic influenza viruses. This level of expertise and the collaborative ethos at its heart has made GISRS an exemplar of how public health agencies worldwide can come together to address global threats to human health and well-being.

In 2017 – 65 years after its founding – discussions were held on how best to mark such an achievement. The long history of GISRS is paved with the tireless efforts of countless dedicated scientists working in developed and developing countries alike – some working in state-of-the-art facilities while others have access to only the most basic equipment. The world owes a debt of gratitude to all those generations of scientists past and present who worked, and continue to work, to make the world a safer place and this book pays homage to them all.

But this book also looks to the future. For as we look back upon and celebrate the successes of the first 65 years of GISRS we must also be mindful that science and history tell us that the next major threat may be just around the corner. For as long as influenza viruses continue to evolve and cause human suffering and economic hardship through seasonal epidemics, sporadic zoonotic infections and highly unpredictable pandemics, GISRS will continue to work to protect individuals and communities and to strengthen global health security in an increasingly interconnected world.

We cannot escape our dangers by recoiling from them.
Winston Churchill

1

Influenza
– a global threat requiring a global response

For hundreds of years of human history influenza has been recognized as a highly contagious and often serious illness, capable of spreading very quickly through affected communities. Signs of illness typically include fever, coughing and often debilitating weakness and physical pain.

But influenza is also a killer. During seasonal "epidemics" it is young children, the elderly and those with chronic underlying conditions who are at greatest risk of dying. Such epidemics thus invariably cause increased levels of mortality, particularly among the elderly, as well as significant societal disruption. Dealing with seasonal influenza epidemics also puts increased pressure on often already overstretched health care services – with potentially serious consequences for the treatment of other life-threatening conditions.

In its even more fearsome "pandemic" form influenza has the potential to wipe out millions of lives in a matter of months – often the lives of the youngest and fittest.

Numerous countries have for many decades perceived influenza as a minor public health threat...the dangers of such complacency are increasingly being recognized.

Despite being a constant threat with truly catastrophic potential, influenza has often remained in the shadow of other national health priorities and has had to compete hard for resources and attention. The reasons for widespread social and political complacency are complex. Most individuals infected by seasonal influenza viruses recover fully after a week or two. In addition, influenza pandemics occur on average only around three times every century.

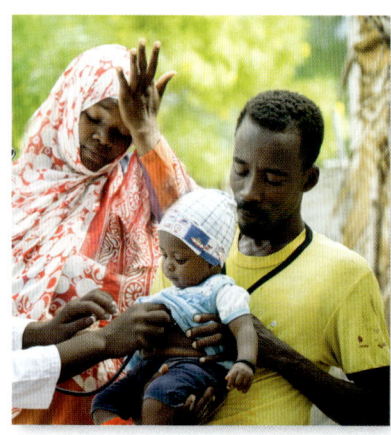

As a result of these and other factors, numerous countries have perceived influenza as a minor public health threat, especially when compared to other infectious diseases such as malaria, hepatitis and HIV/AIDS. The dangers of such complacency in a rapidly changing world are increasingly being recognized.

WHO estimates that around 1 billion cases of seasonal influenza occur annually with around 3–5 million cases of severe illness and 290 000–650 000 deaths.

Seasonal influenza epidemics appear with pronounced regularity during winter and early spring in temperate northern and southern regions of the globe. In tropical and subtropical countries the seasonality of influenza is less well defined. Some of these countries experience one or two epidemic peaks, while in others influenza activity can occur throughout the year. However, as the world becomes ever more connected and the sheer scale of international travel and the movement of people increases, sporadic cases of seasonal influenza or even larger outbreaks can now occur anywhere in the world at any time.

Due to incomplete surveillance and gaps in knowledge, the true global burden of death, disease and economic impact caused each year by these seasonal outbreaks is unknown. However, WHO estimates that around 1 billion cases of seasonal influenza occur annually with around 3–5 million cases of severe illness and 290 000–650 000 deaths. The human, societal and financial costs of this can only be gleaned by looking at settings where robust data collection exists. In the USA, for example, the direct medical costs of seasonal influenza have been estimated at US$ 10.4 billion annually and the total economic burden at US$ 87.1 billion. It is worth bearing in mind that the health, economic and societal costs of these recurring seasonal epidemics are borne by countries each and every year, year after year.

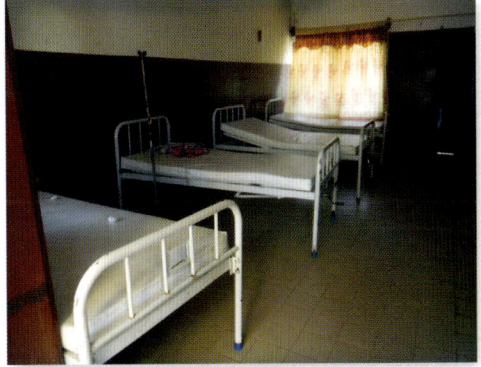

The 1918 "Spanish flu" pandemic remains one of the worst ever global health disasters in human history.

In addition to human seasonal influenza viruses a wide range of animal influenza viruses can also cause influenza in humans. These viruses include the avian influenza subtypes H5N1, H7N9 and H9N2 and the swine influenza subtypes H1N1, H1N2 and H3N2. Such so-called "zoonotic" infections normally only arise through direct contact with infected animals or contaminated environments. Although they occur only sporadically, any case of zoonotic infection is a serious public health concern as the possibility always exists that such viruses will adapt to their new human host and acquire the ability to spread rapidly from person to person.

When such a "novel" influenza virus emerges which contains genes from an animal influenza virus and which can spread quickly from person to person, the onset of a human influenza pandemic becomes a very real possibility. As at least part of such a novel virus is of animal origin then little or no immunity to it will be present in the human

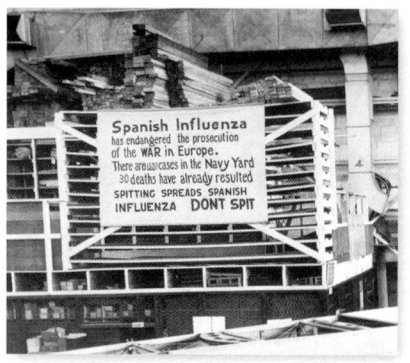

population. In the 100 years since 1917 there have been four such pandemics – in 1918, 1957, 1968 and 2009. None of these pandemics could have been predicted and their impact only became clear in retrospect. In the case of the 1918 "Spanish flu" pandemic, it is currently estimated that at least 50 million deaths occurred globally in the course of only a few months. This figure equates to 3% of the entire population of the world at that time, making it one of the worst ever global health disasters in human history.

Although it is certain that more influenza pandemics will occur in the future, it is impossible to predict when they will happen and which subtypes will cause them. There are currently 18 known subtypes of haemagglutinin and 11 of neuraminidase found in various combinations in birds and other animals.

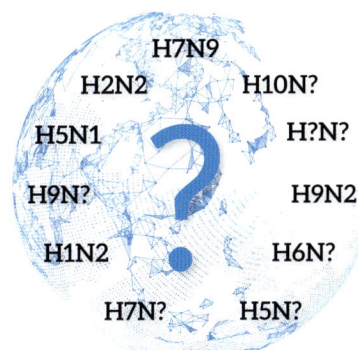

Historically, the only influenza virus subtypes known for certain to have caused a human pandemic have been a combination of H1, H2 or H3 (haemagglutinin) and N1 or N2 (neuraminidase) – such as H1N1 or H2N2. However, the ability of other subtypes to cause a future pandemic is unknown and scientific knowledge is constantly being updated. For example, until 1997 it was widely believed that avian influenza viruses such as H5N1 could not easily attach to the cells lining the human respiratory tract, thus preventing their direct transmission across the species barrier from birds to humans. In 1997 this comforting belief was shattered by the occurrence of 18 human cases of highly pathogenic avian influenza in Hong Kong Special Administrative Region (Hong Kong SAR), China, caused by the H5N1 influenza virus subtype and resulting in six deaths. This event caused a paradigm shift in the international influenza community and the world was forced to think differently about the threat posed by all animal influenza viruses. Since 2003, the H5N1 subtype has caused hundreds of human cases – with about half of them resulting in the death of the individual. In addition, several other avian influenza subtypes have required an emergency-level response from national and international agencies. These include H7N7 viruses in the Netherlands and H7N9 viruses in China, along with other influenza A subtypes such as H5N6 and H9N2.

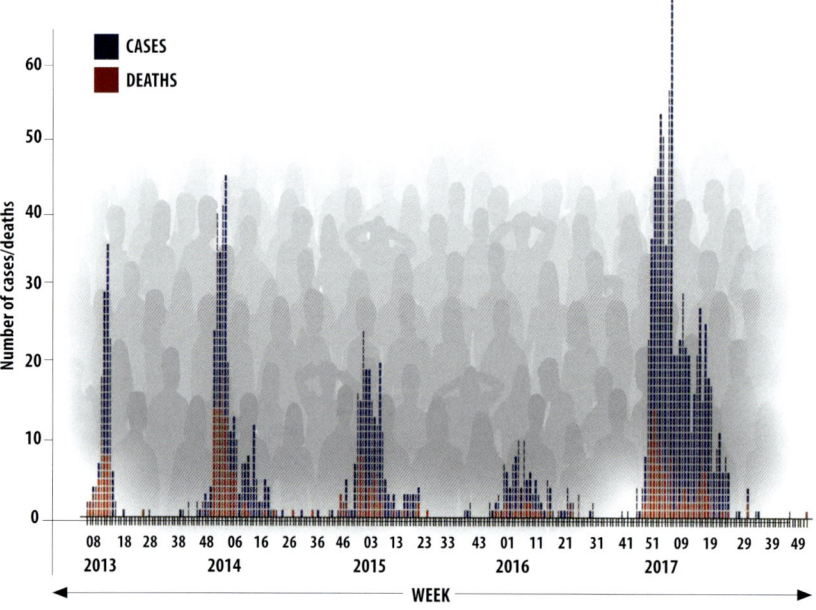

In humans, infection with an avian H7N9 or H5 influenza virus tends to be deadly. As shown above, a total of 1566 laboratory-confirmed human cases of H7N9 infection were reported to WHO during the period 2013–2017. Of these, almost 40% (613 cases) were fatal. Such high levels of fatality are a characteristic feature of zoonotic avian influenza infections, with current WHO estimates of the case-fatality rates of H5N1 infection in humans ranging from 44% to 73% with a cumulative figure of around 53% (453 deaths from 859 confirmed cases).

And seasonal, zoonotic and pandemic influenza are not the only recurring threats to human health and welfare posed by influenza viruses. Influenza outbreaks among animals are both frequent and often devastating for families raising poultry for food, small farms and larger commercial concerns. Although this is particularly the case with well-known highly pathogenic avian influenza viruses such as H5N1, there exists a huge reservoir of other influenza subtypes in both wild and domesticated animals. This poses a constant threat to the livelihood and welfare of people worldwide – typically the poorest and most vulnerable. Furthermore, with a virtually infinite reservoir of influenza viruses circulating in birds, pigs and other animals living in very close proximity to people, the possibility of human infection with an animal influenza virus always exists. There is then a very real risk that such a virus will acquire the ability to spread easily from human to human by the respiratory route thus raising the terrifying spectre of the next human influenza pandemic.

Backyard chicken flocks, live bird markets and industrial poultry farms are all potential settings for outbreaks of avian influenza and the zoonotic transmission of avian influenza viruses to humans. This then brings the subsequent danger of human-to-human transmission and – in the worst-case scenario – a global pandemic. Furthermore, changes in the ecosystem of certain animals, increased global meat consumption, poverty, and political and social unrest can all lead to increased opportunities for animal viruses to cross the species barrier to humans. This requires high levels of alertness by networks conducting influenza surveillance in the veterinary and human health sectors, and close collaboration between these two sectors.

It has been said that influenza is a highly invariable disease caused by a highly variable virus. In fact, the complex biology and ecology of influenza viruses present a never-ending challenge to public health. Because of their incessant evolution – either gradually through the antigenic "drift" of new seasonal viruses or through the sudden antigenic "shift" capable of producing a novel virus with pandemic potential – new antigenic variants of influenza viruses frequently arise in different parts of the world. Without constant vigilance and monitoring, there would be no possibility of detecting the emergence of new influenza viruses early enough to do anything about them – whether epidemic or pandemic. For example, seasonal influenza vaccines would not only fail to be produced in time they could not be produced at all. Similarly, other medical and non-medical interventions, often highly specific to influenza and known to work in times of health emergencies, could almost certainly never be implemented quickly enough to make any difference.

In such an interconnected world, national boundaries are no barrier to contagious disease spread ...

As the world becomes ever more connected, the ease with which millions of people and animals cross national borders every day presents a huge challenge for the public health community. In such an interconnected world, national boundaries are no barrier to contagious disease spread and only a truly international collaboration coordinated at the global level can meet this challenge.

Since 1952, the mission of GISRS has been to provide the platform for the world to collaborate in detecting and responding to seasonal influenza epidemics, sporadic zoonotic infections and highly unpredictable pandemics. During this time, GISRS has repeatedly demonstrated its ability to quickly recognize emerging situations and to rapidly and flexibly respond to a broad range of threats and challenges. On numerous occasions, including the 1957, 1968 and 2009 influenza pandemics, and the re-emergence of H1N1 influenza viruses in 1977, rapid actions have been taken to mount a global public health response to these threats.

When it comes to influenza – seasonal or pandemic – the world cannot afford to sit back and wait. Through its proactive and unceasing efforts each year to track the emergence and spread of influenza viruses, monitor their impact on human health and ensure the open sharing of viruses and related data, GISRS has for 65 years been at the forefront of the world's fight against influenza and other dangerous respiratory viruses.

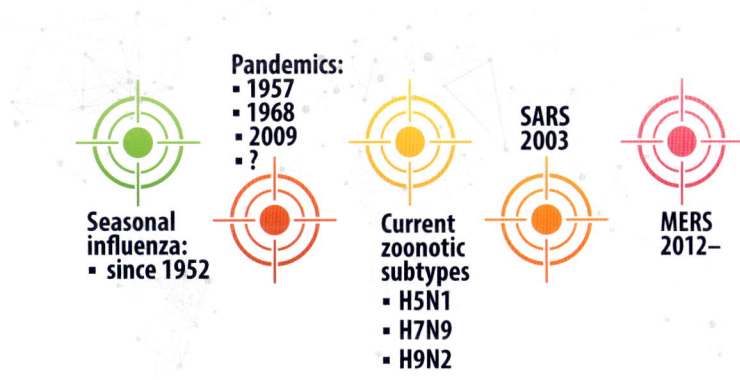

MERS = Middle East respiratory syndrome; SARS = severe acute respiratory syndrome.

1918–1947
– aftermath of a devastating pandemic

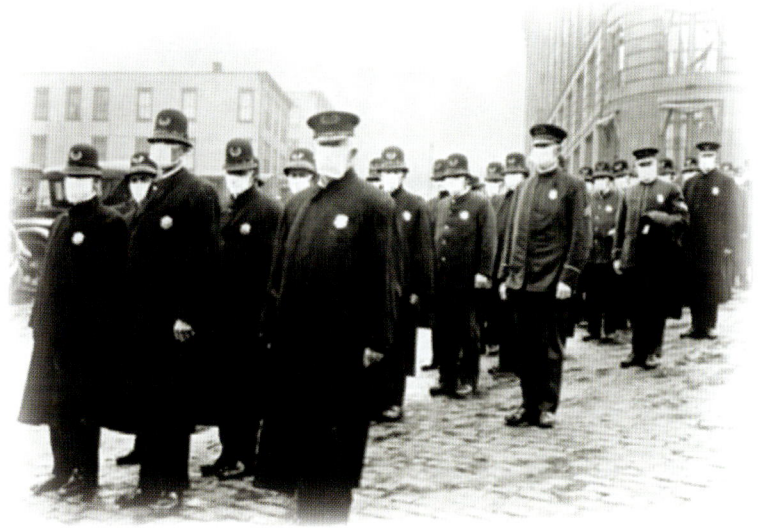

In 1918 the catastrophic Spanish flu pandemic alerted the world to the deadly threat to humankind posed by influenza. Nevertheless, it would require almost 30 years of scientific research and discovery – much of it taking place against a background of international conflict and upheaval – before the possibility of mounting a united global effort against this threat became a reality.

Just over a decade after the 1918 Spanish flu pandemic, researchers succeeded in isolating influenza viruses – first from pigs in 1931 and then from humans in 1933. Prior to these discoveries it was believed that the causative agent of influenza was the bacterium *Haemophilus influenzae*. Although the concept of a virus pathogen distinct from bacteria had been demonstrated in plants at the end of the nineteenth century it was not until the early twentieth century that laboratory methods finally became available to isolate and grow viruses from animals and humans.

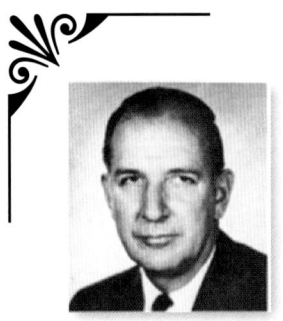

SWINE INFLUENZA

I. EXPERIMENTAL TRANSMISSION AND PATHOLOGY

BY RICHARD E. SHOPE, M.D.

(From the Department of Animal Pathology of The Rockefeller Institute for Medical Research, Princeton, N. J.)

II. A HEMOPHILIC BACILLUS FROM THE RESPIRATORY TRACT OF INFECTED SWINE

BY PAUL A. LEWIS, M.D., AND RICHARD E. SHOPE, M.D.

(From the Department of Animal Pathology of The Rockefeller Institute for Medical Research, Princeton, N. J.)

III. FILTRATION EXPERIMENTS AND ETIOLOGY

BY RICHARD E. SHOPE, M.D.

(From the Department of Animal Pathology of The Rockefeller Institute for Medical Research, Princeton, N. J.)

In 1931, during an outbreak of swine influenza in the Midwestern USA, Dr Richard Shope inoculated healthy pigs with a filtrate of respiratory secretions collected from ill pigs. This was the first experimental transmission of an influenza virus and resulted in illness in the previously healthy pigs. The symptoms produced in pigs were found to be more severe when the virus-containing filtrate was combined with Haemophilus influenzae suis, a bacterium often found in the respiratory tract of pigs with influenza-like symptoms. Dr Shope also demonstrated that people who had experienced the Spanish flu pandemic in 1918 had antibodies to the swine influenza virus.

Even with the technology available at that time it was apparent to early researchers that these swine and human influenza viruses were closely related to each other. As these were the first "type" of influenza virus discovered they were classified as type A influenza viruses. Subsequently, in the course of an influenza outbreak in New York in 1940, an influenza virus was isolated which was clearly distinct from the type A viruses and this became the first type B influenza virus. This nomenclature remains unchanged to this day.

In 1933, researchers inoculated ferrets with filtered fluid obtained from the respiratory secretions of patients with influenza-like illness. The ferrets developed clinical signs such as fever and respiratory symptoms resembling those of human influenza. This was thus the first successful isolation of human influenza viruses.

THE LANCET

Volume 222: 8 July, 1933

A VIRUS OBTAINED FROM INFLUENZA PATIENTS

By Wilson Smith, M.D. Manch.
C. H. Andrewes, M.D. Lond.
AND
P. P. Laidlaw, B.Chir. Camb., F.R.S.

(From the National Institute for Medical Research, Farm Laboratories, Mill Hill)

The epidemic of influenza at the beginning of 1933 afforded an opportunity of making an experimental study of this disease, the results of which are here embodied in a preliminary communication. Throat-washings were obtained from a number of patients as early as possible after the onset of definite symptoms. On the assumption that the ætiological agent of influenza was probably a filtrable virus the throat-washings were filtered before use through a membrane impermeable to bacteria. The filtrates, proved to be bacteriologically sterile, were used in attempts to infect many different species. All such attempts were entirely unsuccessful until the ferret was used and the first success was only secured towards the close of the epidemic.

Developing an influenza vaccine quickly became an urgent priority…

Most of the researchers working on influenza during those early years had witnessed first-hand the devastating effects of the Spanish flu pandemic and they all agreed that such a global pandemic could arise again. In addition, the severity of annual seasonal influenza epidemics was beginning to be recognized. Such insights naturally led to thoughts of developing a vaccine that could offer protection against influenza viruses, and preliminary experiments soon followed. Developing an influenza vaccine quickly became an urgent priority, including for the United States military following huge losses due to pandemic influenza among its soldiers during World War I and its immediate aftermath.

Shortly after the isolation of human influenza viruses in 1933, two advances were made which still form the basis of influenza vaccine production today. The first was the successful adaptation of candidate influenza vaccine viruses to grow in large numbers in embryonated hens' eggs. The second was the discovery that the natural ability of influenza viruses to cause red blood cells to clump together (haemagglutinate) in test tubes was inhibited if well-matched antibodies to them were also present in the mixture. This procedure was named the "haemagglutination inhibition test" and to this day it remains a vital tool for characterizing influenza viruses. Together, these two discoveries allow for emerging viruses which are not inhibited by existing human antibodies to be identified and then grown on an industrial scale for inclusion in vaccines.

Researchers were also able to demonstrate that seasonal influenza viruses exhibited different antigenic characteristics from year to year – even if they belonged to the same type. This was a watershed moment in the history of influenza vaccination. It became clear that during the replication of influenza viruses in host cells, genetic mutations could occur which resulted in changes, particularly in the two surface proteins (haemagglutinin and neuraminidase) which are the principal targets of human immune responses. This type of gradual evolutionary pathway became known as "antigenic drift". In this scenario, antibodies derived from a previous infection or from prior vaccination may no longer recognize drifted viruses, which can then escape attack by the individual's immune system and cause illness.

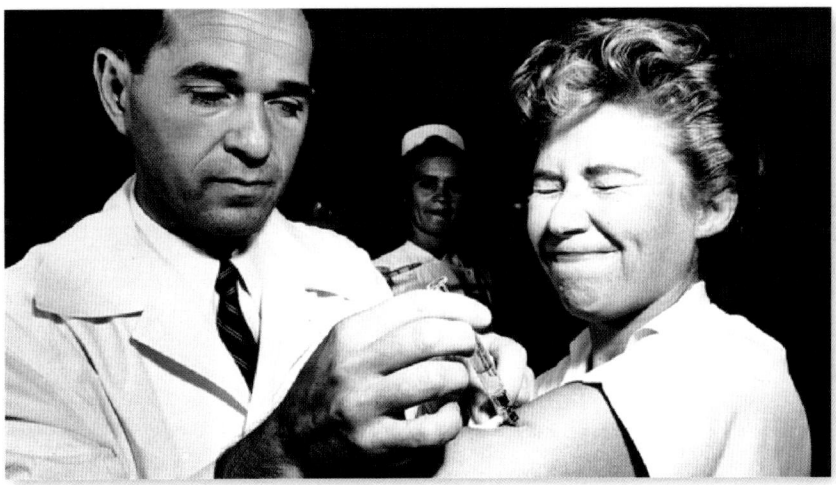

Because of constant antigenic drift, the optimal set of viruses to include in a seasonal influenza vaccine changes over time, requiring their frequent updating and annual administration.

Shortly after the development of the first efficacious influenza vaccine in 1943, licensed vaccines were approved in the USA – first for military use and then later for civilian use. However, encouraging early success was soon followed by a major disappointment in the 1946–47 influenza season when a large vaccine trial turned out to be a complete failure. Despite being properly immunized with preparations that had shown good results in previous studies, the individuals in this new trial acquired little or no protection at all.

The emergence of such a distinct new variant immediately stirred memories of the devastation of 1918...

The emergence of a distinct new variant that was capable of rendering the newly developed vaccine ineffective immediately stirred memories of the devastation of 1918 and for many years it was wrongly believed that the 1947 virus had undergone a process known as "antigenic shift". Compared to the much more gradual seasonal antigenic drift, antigenic shift involves the swapping of genes between different human and animal influenza viruses. Antigenic shift is the process which can lead to the emergence of influenza viruses with the potential to cause a pandemic.

Recognition of the possibility of antigenic shift further underlined the crucial need for continual surveillance of influenza viruses, their biological characteristics, their epidemiological spread and the clinical illnesses they cause. Given the global spread of influenza viruses, it was quickly realized that this could only be achieved by establishing an international network of laboratories to collect and characterize circulating influenza viruses and to freely exchange virus isolates, clinical specimens and related epidemiological, virological and other data. Only through such international collaboration would it be possible to produce an effective seasonal influenza vaccine each year while also remaining vigilant against emerging strains with pandemic potential.

WHO.IC/97

13 August 1947

INTERNATIONAL COLLABORATION
IN THE INFLUENZA FIELD

Note by Dr. C. H. Andrewes, National Institute
for Medical Research, Hampstead, London

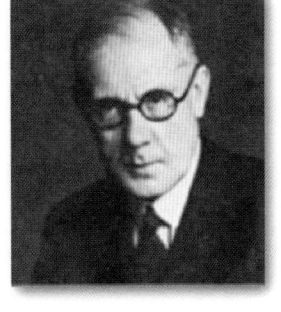

For the last decade or more, influenza has caused considerable economic loss to nearly all countries; it has not, however, been the alarming, killing disease that it was in 1918–1919. It is generally believed that the influenza virus is a particularly labile one apt to produce mutant strains and that one or more such mutants caused the 1918–1919 pandemic. So far as we know, the virus may at any time produce another such mutant, and again kill its millions.

Existing vaccines would be unlikely to be very effective against this, if at all. Some effect of antibiotics against secondary bacterial invaders is to be hoped for, but drug-resistant bacteria might quickly become prevalent.

To avert "another 1918", we need, most of all, to gain understanding of the epidemiology of the influenza of these times, in the hope of learning, amongst other things, about the occurrence of mutants and their spread.

Though some striking successes in vaccination against influenza have been reported from the United States of America, last winter's results have been disappointing, perhaps because 1947 strains have been antigenically remote from the strain used for the vaccine. One might perhaps hope to isolate a strain from the beginning of an epidemic, adapt it to growth in fertile eggs and produce a vaccine in time to be of use before the epidemic is over.

In practice, there is not nearly enough time to do this within one country. But if it could be shown that a new – and especially a lethal – strain was spreading from country to country, the vaccine might be produced in time to protect countries yet unattacked. The above arguments seem to show that many problems concerning influenza can be solved only by international collaboration, such as could be fostered by the World Health Organization.

The beginning is the most important part of the work.
                                             Plato

1947–1952
– the birth of GISRS

In 1946 the United Nations established an Interim Commission specifically tasked with guiding the establishment and early activities of the soon-to-be-inaugurated World Health Organization (WHO). By this time, the need for international collaboration in influenza monitoring and response activities was already a recognized priority in global public health. Influenza was thus one of the first diseases in history to be officially acknowledged as a global threat requiring a global response, with the idea of an international network of collaborating influenza laboratories predating the coming into force of the WHO Constitution in 1948.

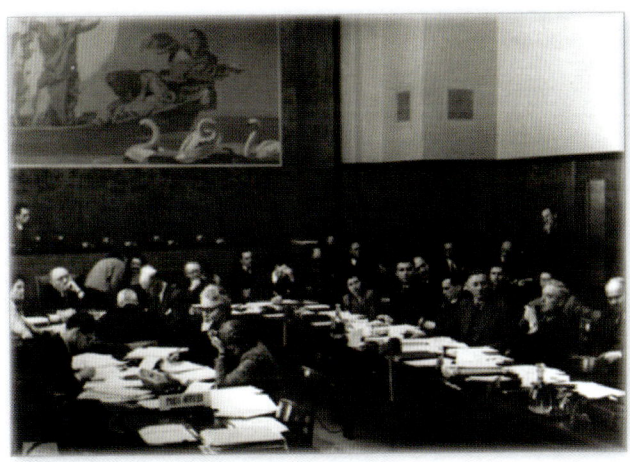

Among the deliberations of the Interim Commission established in 1946 was the need for international collaboration in influenza monitoring and response activities.

On 3 April 1947, during the third session of the Interim Commission, Dr C van den Berg, the Representative from the Netherlands, proposed the setting up of a committee on influenza, noting that *the outbreak of an influenza pandemic in the nearest future should on no account be considered an imaginary danger*. At the Fourth International Congress for Microbiology, held in Copenhagen in July 1947, a panel of elected members submitted suggestions to the Interim Commission for promoting international collaboration in this field.

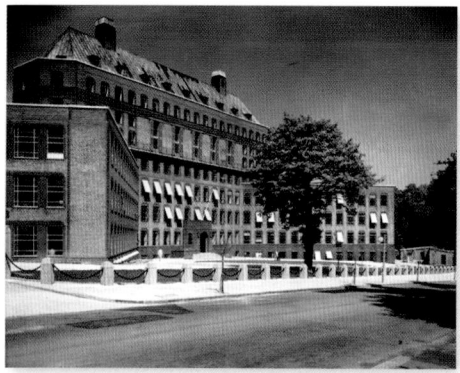

The famous Mill Hill building in North London became home to the World Influenza Centre from 1949 until it moved to the new Francis Crick Institute in central London in 2016. As the site for the initial identification of human influenza viruses in 1933 and related pioneering research, Mill Hill was considered the natural choice and ideal location for such an endeavour.

In July 1948, three months after the WHO Constitution entered into force, members of the 10th meeting of the Committee on the Programme of WHO formally approved the establishment and funding of a "World Influenza Centre" under the aegis of the National Institute for Medical Research in London. Occurring 30 years after the Spanish flu pandemic, this landmark event was one of a number of important steps taken by scientists and senior public health experts to ensure that the world would never again be so unprepared for the onset of a deadly influenza pandemic.

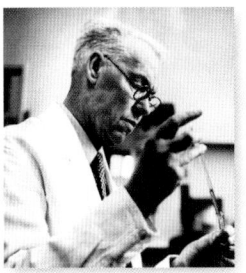 Dr Christopher Howard Andrewes was part of the team that first studied human influenza viruses in 1933 and served as the head of the Division of Bacteriology and Virus Research within the National Institute for Medical Research where he became the first director of the World Influenza Centre.

The primary tasks of the World Influenza Centre were:

- to establish a network of laboratories to collect and characterize influenza viruses, and disseminate the outcomes of their investigations;
- to collect, characterize and preserve influenza virus strains from ongoing outbreaks and distribute samples and reagents to relevant laboratories;
- to provide laboratory training to visiting staff.

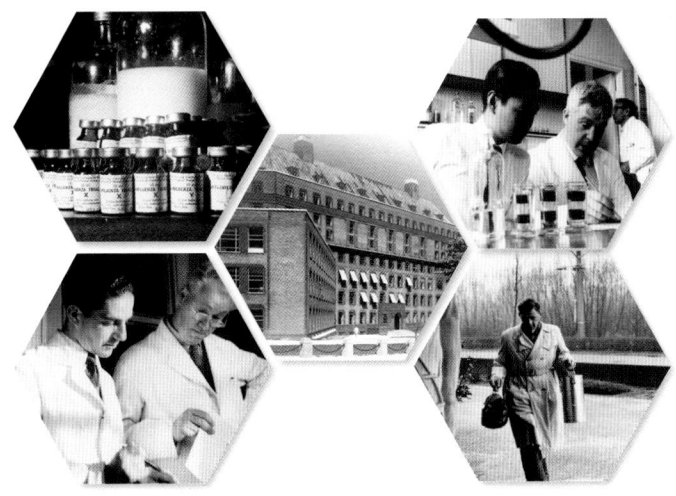

In early 1949, the Executive Board of WHO requested Member States to provide information on circulating influenza viruses. This included information on their clinical impact, on morbidity and mortality among specific age groups, and on the actions that could be taken to control the disease. Although a number of countries already had national influenza surveillance systems in place and were reporting data to WHO, it soon became clear that such surveillance needed to be coordinated internationally and expanded to parts of the world not yet covered. In September 1951, Dr Andrewes called an informal meeting on influenza in order to discuss *the operation of the present network of influenza laboratories throughout the world, under the aegis of WHO and the need for international coordination of research in the field of influenza, and the points which a WHO expert committee might most usefully consider.*

The subsequently established WHO Expert Committee on Influenza met for the first time in 1952. This event is now widely regarded as signalling the start of global influenza surveillance and response activities under the coordination of WHO – and thus the birth of what would eventually become GISRS. In its first report in April 1953, the Committee summarized the available scientific knowledge regarding influenza and presented its recommendations on the collection and sharing of influenza surveillance data. In its conclusions, the Committee pointed out three activity areas in particular that would benefit from the active participation and coordination capabilities of WHO:

- disseminating information on the prevention and control of influenza;
- training of professionals to carry out laboratory and epidemiological investigations;
- supplying diagnostic materials free of charge to laboratories participating in influenza surveillance activities.

EXPERT COMMITTEE ON INFLUENZA

First Session

Geneva, 8-12 September 1952

Members:

Dr. C. H. Andrewes, World Influenza Centre of the World Health Organization; Deputy Director, National Institute for Medical Research, Mill Hill, London, United Kingdom of Great Britain and Northern Ireland

Professor I. Archetti, Istituto Superiore di Sanità, Rome, Italy

Dr. Dorland J. Davis, Executive Secretary, Influenza Information Center, National Institutes of Health (US Public Health Service), Bethesda, Md., USA

Dr. M. R. Hilleman, Chief, Diagnostic and Respiratory Research Sections, Department of Virus and Rickettsial Diseases, Army Medical Service Graduate School, Washington, D.C., USA

Professeur P. Lépine, Chef du Service des Virus, Institut Pasteur, Paris, France (*Chairman*)

Professor T. P. Magill, Strain Study Center for the Americas, Department of Microbiology and Immunology, State University Medical Center at New York College of Medicine, Brooklyn, N.Y., USA (*Vice-Chairman*)

Dr. Preben von Magnus, Chief of Laboratory, Statens Seruminstitut, Copenhagen, Denmark

Dr. J. Mulder, Professor of Medicine, University Medical Clinic, Leyden, Netherlands

Professor C. H. Stuart-Harris, University Department of Medicine, The Royal Hospital, Sheffield, United Kingdom of Great Britain and Northern Ireland (*Rapporteur*)

WORLD HEALTH ORGANIZATION
TECHNICAL REPORT SERIES

No. 64

EXPERT COMMITTEE ON INFLUENZA

First Report

	Page
1. Introduction	3
2. Grouping of the influenza viruses	4
3. Importance of continued study of the influenza virus antigens	5
4. Methods of comparing and typing strains	6
5. Designation of newly isolated influenza virus strains	7
6. Methods of collection and distribution of specimens	7
7. Recommendations for standard diagnostic procedures	9
8. Influenza virus vaccines	10
9. Collection and distribution of epidemiological information regarding influenza	13
10. Control measures against severe epidemics of influenza	15
11. Therapeutic measures in influenza	16
12. Training of laboratory workers	17
13. Exchange of publications	17
14. General conclusions	17
Annex 1. Methods of preparation of antisera for the comparison and typing of strains of influenza virus	20
Annex 2. Techniques recommended for standard diagnostic procedures	24

The 1952 meeting of the nine WHO-appointed influenza experts shown above and its resulting report signalled the beginning of what was to become GISRS.

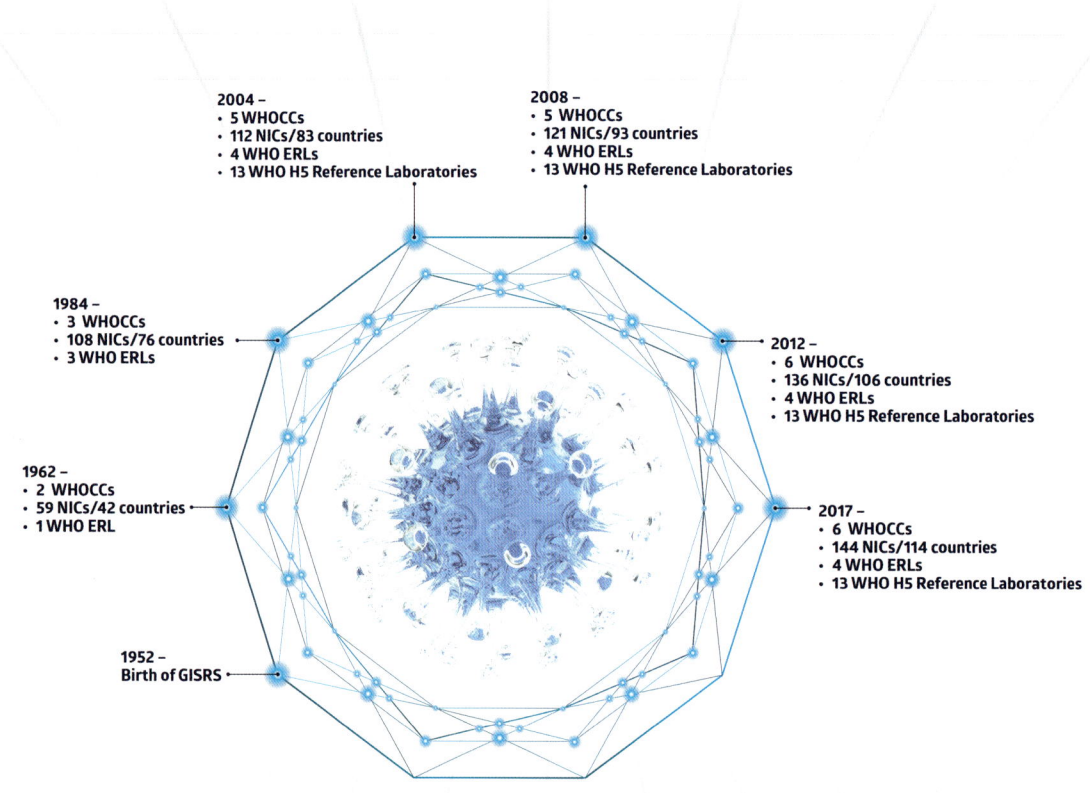

NIC = National Influenza Centre; WHOCC = WHO Collaborating Centre; WHO ERL = WHO Essential Regulatory Laboratory.

For almost 60 years (1952–2011) this WHO-coordinated initiative was known as the Global Influenza Surveillance Network (GISN). In 2003, the re-emergence of human cases of infection with avian H5N1 influenza viruses was quickly followed by the rapid spread of the virus among domesticated birds in several countries in Asia. This led to calls by WHO Member States for a mechanism to facilitate not only the rapid, systematic and timely sharing of influenza viruses with pandemic potential, but also fairer and more efficient access by all countries to the resulting benefits, notably pandemic vaccines. Following four years of formal and informal discussions among WHO Member States and a broad and diverse group of stakeholders, the landmark Pandemic Influenza Preparedness Framework for the Sharing of Influenza Viruses and Access to Vaccines and other Benefits (PIP Framework) was adopted by the Sixty-fourth World Health Assembly on 24 May 2011. Among other changes, Member States agreed to rename GISN to better reflect its expanded scope covering both surveillance and response, and as a result the name "Global Influenza Surveillance and Response System (GISRS)" has been used ever since.

GISRS
– a public health resource for the world

Since its foundation in 1952, GISRS has undergone a remarkable expansion in both its global reach and range of core activities. Originally known as the "Global Influenza Surveillance Network", the new initiative consisted principally of the World Influenza Centre in London and 21 national laboratories that were formally recognized as National Influenza Centres (NICs). Each of the six WHO regions had at least one such laboratory at that time sending influenza surveillance information to the World Influenza Centre. Given that the impetus for the establishment of an influenza surveillance network came primarily from European scientists it is not surprising that 11 of the original 21 NICs were located in countries of the WHO European Region.

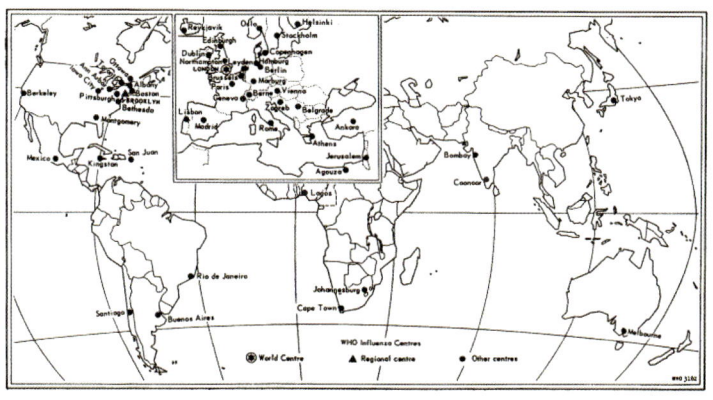

By 1953, the surveillance network consisted of 54 NICs in 42 countries providing data to the World Influenza Centre. During these early years around half of all NICs were located in Europe and a fifth in North America. By contrast, in the entire WHO South-East Asia Region there were only two, both situated in India.

However, growing awareness that influenza was a global issue requiring a global approach continued to drive the geographical expansion of laboratory coverage, and continues to do so today. By 1969, GISRS included 80 NICs in 55 countries, areas or territories, with this number increasing to 101 in 1979 and 110 in 2002. By 2017, 65 years after its foundation, GISRS had grown to encompass more than 150 NICs and other laboratories in 114 WHO Member States and territories.

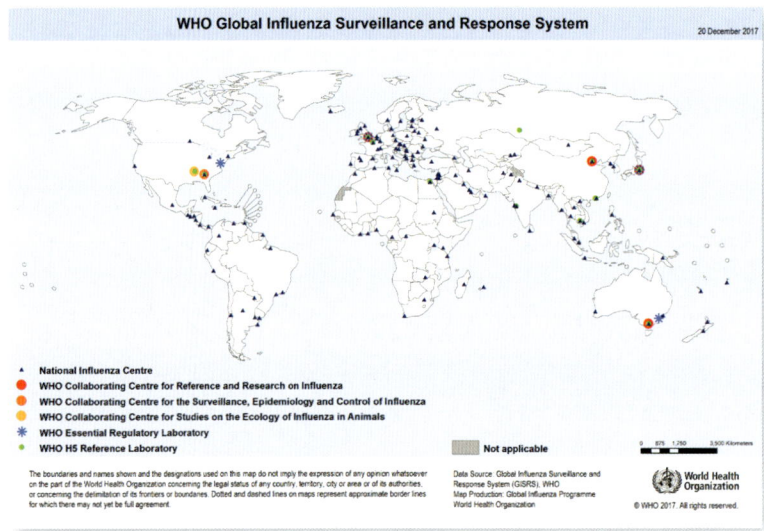

Today, GISRS spans the entire world, with the number of WHO-recognized NICs increasing in all six WHO regions. As of January 2017, GISRS consisted of 144 NICs in 114 countries, six WHO Collaborating Centres (WHOCCs), 13 WHO H5 Reference Laboratories and four WHO Essential Regulatory Laboratories (ERLs).

NICs are the backbone of GISRS...

NICs are the backbone of GISRS and from its very beginning have worked to protect national and global health by contributing the virus isolates and related virological and epidemiological data needed to update seasonal influenza vaccines. At the same time, NICs also act as a frontline global alert mechanism for the emergence of influenza viruses that have the potential to cause a human pandemic. Within countries, the NIC is thus likely to be the primary source of expertise in the laboratory surveillance of influenza epidemics and pandemics. Consequently, the triggering of many of the interventions described in national influenza preparedness plans will depend upon the effective functioning of the NIC.

In addition to performing laboratory analyses, NICs also gather data and information on the geographical spread and impact of influenza in their countries. They then report their findings regularly – often weekly – to national authorities, regional agencies and the centralized WHO FluNet database. NICs also send representative clinical specimens or virus isolates to one of the six WHOCCs, especially isolates which display unusual or atypical characteristics.

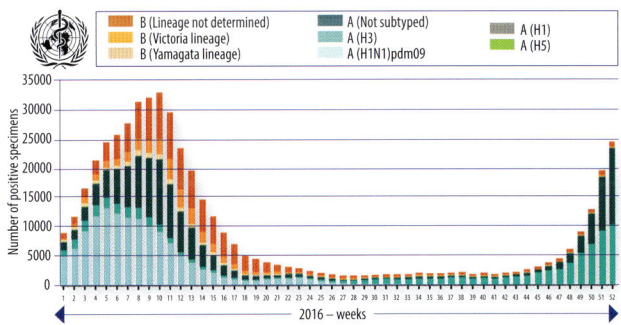

Through these and other efforts, NICs work year-round to provide a real-time and continually updated picture of the national influenza situation, which is then used to inform scientific risk assessments and to guide appropriate public health measures in countries.

Expansion of the WHO FluNet database – NICs routinely report on the number of clinical specimens tested each week and on the number testing positive for influenza. This allows for an indication to be given of the most commonly circulating influenza virus types and subtypes. In 1997, the first year of its operation, WHO FluNet was notified of approximately 12 000 positive specimens. By 2016, as shown above, the annual figure was approaching half a million, equating to around one in every six of the 3 million specimens tested that year.

WHOCCs are another fundamental GISRS component ...

And NICs are only part of an ever-expanding GISRS. Following the early realization that the workload of the World Influenza Centre in London would be substantial and likely to rapidly increase, other influenza reference laboratories around the world began to be officially designated as WHOCCs on influenza. WHOCCs are another long-established and essential component of GISRS, providing much-needed capacity and high levels of expertise, cooperation and assistance. These institutions are financially supported by their governments and/or other entities for all activities related to meeting their GISRS responsibilities. Many of the scientists working in the WHOCCs have long-standing international reputations in the field of influenza, and have authored publications in high-profile international journals. As the history and development of each WHOCC differ considerably, each brings its own specialist capabilities and individual strengths, in addition to a common set of core capacities.

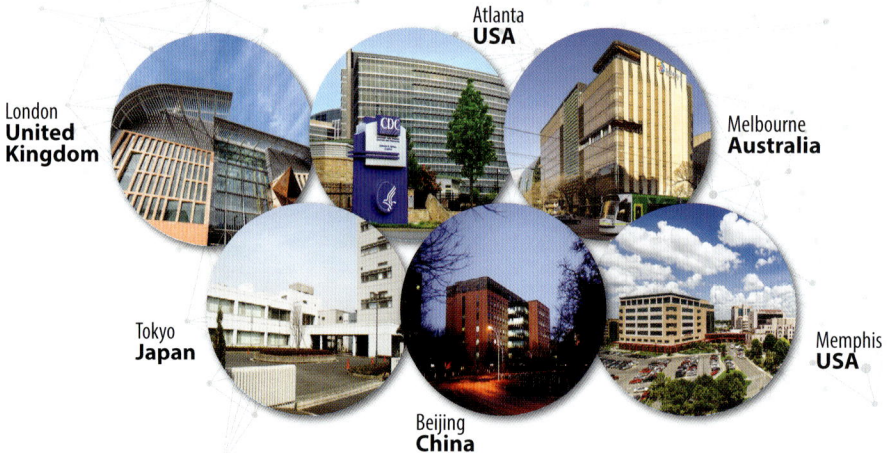

Starting in 1956, five additional WHOCCs have now joined forces with the World Influenza Centre in London to progressively strengthen the activities of GISRS. Following the move of the World Influenza Centre to the Francis Crick Institute in 2016 these six WHOCCs are housed in the following institutions: the Francis Crick Institute, London, United Kingdom (since 2016); the Centers for Disease Control and Prevention, Atlanta, Georgia, USA (1956); the Victorian Infectious Diseases Reference Laboratory, Melbourne, Australia (1992); the National Institute of Infectious Diseases, Tokyo, Japan (1993); the Chinese Center for Disease Control and Prevention, Beijing, China (2010); and the St Jude Children's Research Hospital, Memphis, Tennessee, USA (1975).

WHO ERLs play a key role...

In addition to NICs and WHOCCs there are other types of institutions which make up GISRS. These include four WHO ERLs that specialize in the standardization and quality testing of seasonal and pandemic influenza vaccines. Some of these laboratories prepare and distribute the "high-growth reassortant" viruses required for vaccine production along with reagents for testing the quality, specificity and antigen content of such vaccines. Furthermore, some WHO ERLs ensure the collection of sera from individuals of different ages who have been immunized with the vaccine used during the preceding season. Serological methods are then used to determine how well influenza-specific antibodies in these sera recognize currently circulating influenza viruses. This is a very important step in evaluating the need to update the WHO recommendations on the composition of seasonal influenza vaccines.

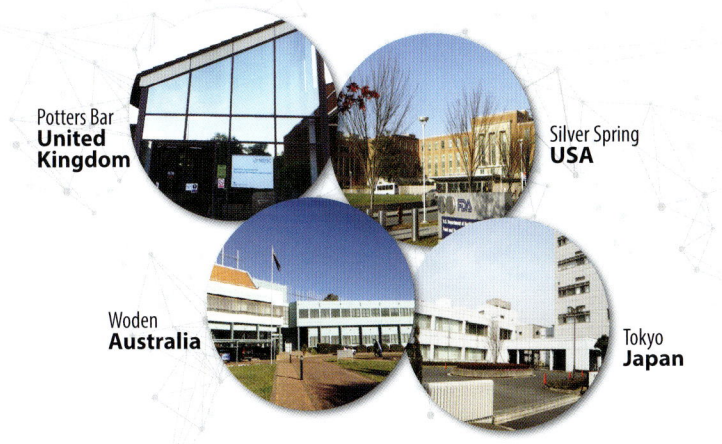

The four WHO ERLs are housed in the following institutions: the National Institute for Biological Standards and Control, Potters Bar, United Kingdom; the Food and Drug Administration, Silver Spring, Maryland, USA; the Therapeutic Goods Administration, Woden, Australian Capital Territory, Australia; and the National Institute of Infectious Diseases, Tokyo, Japan.

In 2004, a number of specialized laboratories were invited to become WHO H5 Reference Laboratories as an ad hoc part of GISRS.

In 2004, the re-emergence of human cases of infection with highly pathogenic avian H5N1 influenza viruses in South-East Asia and elsewhere highlighted the clear need for the participation of laboratories with the ability to promptly and reliably detect influenza viruses at the animal–human interface, and the capabilities needed to work safely with such highly dangerous pathogens. As many NICs at that time did not possess such capabilities, a number of specialized laboratories were invited to become WHO H5 Reference Laboratories as an ad hoc part of GISRS. At present, there are 13 such laboratories playing a vital role in GISRS activities, many of which are located within a WHOCC or NIC. Thanks to national capacity-building gains in recent years, the need for support from WHO H5 Reference laboratories has decreased in many countries. This welcome trend is increasingly leading to the more integrated and enhanced ability of countries to handle dangerous pathogens as part of a wide range of routine national influenza activities.

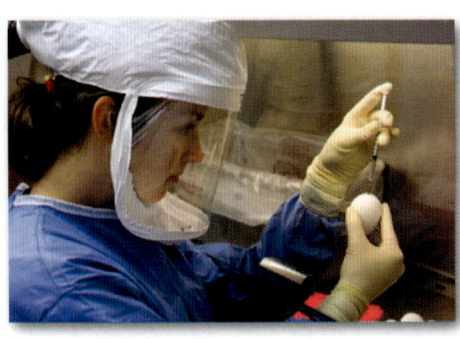

In addition to the four types of GISRS entities outlined above, numerous epidemiological, academic research and other institutions working at local, national, regional or global level also make considerable contributions to the work of GISRS. Although not formally affiliated with WHO or GISRS, such institutions nevertheless play a key role in a broad range of GISRS activities, such as the preparation of specific reagents or high-growth reassortant viruses, the provision of training opportunities, the sharing of data and the furthering of scientific understanding of influenza. The numerous activities conducted by NICs, WHOCCs, WHO ERLs and WHO H5 Reference Laboratories, working together under the umbrella of GISRS, generate an enormous volume of data and other information for use in academic research. Over the years, this has led to the publication of countless scientific research papers and other communications.

In 2008, NICs collectively tested around half a million specimens for influenza viruses – by 2017 this figure had reached almost 3.5 million.

The historical expansion of GISRS has been matched by a corresponding increase in the scale of its surveillance activities and other public health functions. Influenza surveillance typically begins with a doctor recognizing the need to determine the cause of a patient's illness. A clinical sample taken from the patient – usually a nasal and/or throat swab – is then sent for laboratory identification of the causative influenza virus or other pathogen.

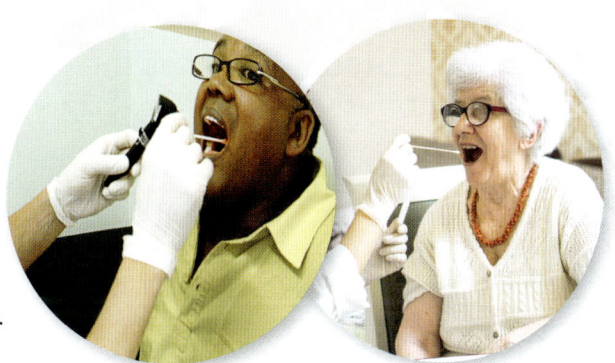

In many countries an established "sentinel" network of doctors regularly and routinely collects samples from patients presenting with clinical symptoms consistent with influenza or an influenza-like illness.

The clinical specimens obtained are then analysed in more detail – either directly by the NIC or after the forwarding of specimens or influenza isolates by other specialized laboratories in the national network. Each year, GISRS provides NICs with a reagent kit prepared by the WHOCC, Atlanta that allows them to distinguish between influenza types A and B, and to identify the virus subtype or lineage. In recent years, the repertoire of laboratory tests used by NICs for the detection and characterization of influenza viruses has expanded significantly. Along with the traditionally used laboratory tests, a wide range of molecular assays, next-generation genetic analysis and other advanced techniques are now routinely performed by many NICs. In 2008, NICs collectively tested around half a million specimens for influenza viruses. During the 2009 H1N1 pandemic, this figure exceeded 2 million, with 26 000 clinical specimens and virus isolates forwarded to WHOCCs for further detailed analysis. In 2017, the total number of specimens tested by NICs in a single year reached almost 3.5 million.

Each year, the six WHOCCs receive thousands of clinical specimens and influenza virus isolates from NICs for highly advanced analysis and characterization. This currently includes detailed antigenic testing based on the ability of viruses to agglutinate red blood cells and on how efficiently they are neutralized by antibodies to previously circulating viruses. WHOCCs then report back their findings to the originating NIC. This vital step in the surveillance process allows countries to better understand the virological characteristics of viruses circulating in their population. Based on this and other information received from the WHOCCs, the NIC can update its diagnostic and analytical laboratory procedures accordingly.

Advanced sequencing technology has the potential to bring about a revolution in global influenza surveillance and response activities.

WHOCCs and many NICs also routinely sequence viral genes, primarily those which code for the haemagglutinin and neuraminidase surface proteins. Viruses with properties of interest from many different parts of the world can now be exchanged and characterized in minute detail to allow for careful and continual monitoring of their epidemiological impact and spread. As ever more-advanced sequencing technology becomes available, the entire genome of an increasing number of viruses can be rapidly sequenced. Such advances have the potential to bring about a revolution in global influenza surveillance and response activities.

From its earliest beginnings, GISRS has continually grown and evolved, and is today almost unrecognizable in terms of both its global reach and extent of its activities compared to the European-centred network from which it first sprang. Although many of the remarkable technological advances that have taken place could not have been envisaged by its early pioneers, the spirit of partnership that underlies GISRS, its openness to new collaborations and technologies, and its determination to monitor and respond to the threat of influenza remain unchanged. GISRS will continue to use the wealth of virus isolates, virological and epidemiological data, and other information generated by its activities to drive forward the range of crucially important and recurring global public health and health security activities described in subsequent chapters of this book.

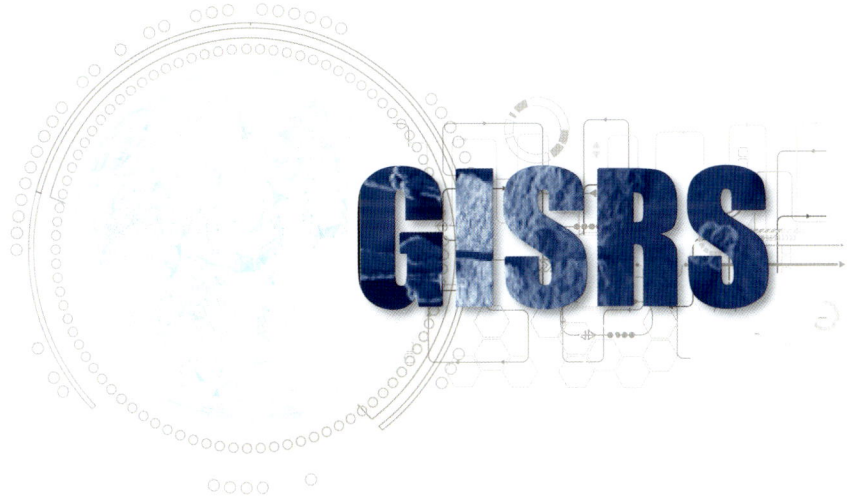

5

From WHO recommendations to seasonal influenza vaccine production

The issuing of WHO recommendations on the optimal composition of seasonal influenza vaccines is one of the fundamental public health outcomes of GISRS activities. In 1953, the first report of the WHO Expert Committee on Influenza included a chapter on influenza vaccines. It was quickly recognized that any vaccine virus must be closely related to the virus against which protection is desired. The report went on to say that this could be achieved either by using a mixture of all known viruses or by including one or two virus strains responsible for the most recent outbreaks. However, due to the rapid evolution of influenza viruses, the report concluded that *in either case, there is a risk that the forthcoming epidemic may in fact be caused by an antigenic variant not represented in the vaccine.*

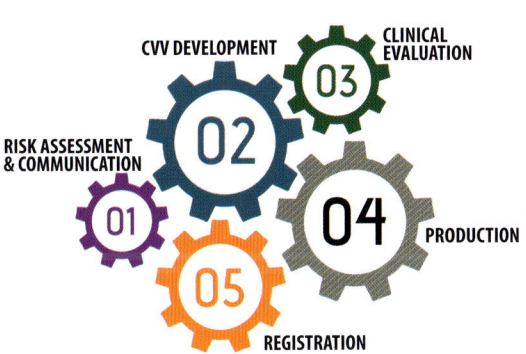

The virological and epidemiological information generated through GISRS surveillance activities is the key to the development and production of influenza vaccines. Ensuring the best possible chance of producing effective and well-matched seasonal influenza vaccines each year requires open, intensive and highly technical collaboration with vaccine manufacturers and other partners. This collaboration has led over many years to the development of an enduring and successful model of public–private partnership and cooperation that is unparalleled in any other sphere of public health.

The first formal WHO recommendations on influenza vaccine composition were issued in 1971. Since 1998, separate recommendations have been issued each year in February and September for the northern and southern hemispheres, respectively. In both cases, these recommendations are made around 8 months prior to the upcoming influenza season as this is currently the minimum time required to manufacture, distribute and administer the required quantities of seasonal influenza vaccines. As the recommendations for the upcoming season must often be made before the current season has ended, this requires considerable skill in analysing complex datasets to predict the most likely course of virus evolution and spread. This and the long lead-in time required for influenza vaccine manufacture unavoidably means that seasonal influenza vaccine production is highly challenging and must be carried out under severe time pressures.

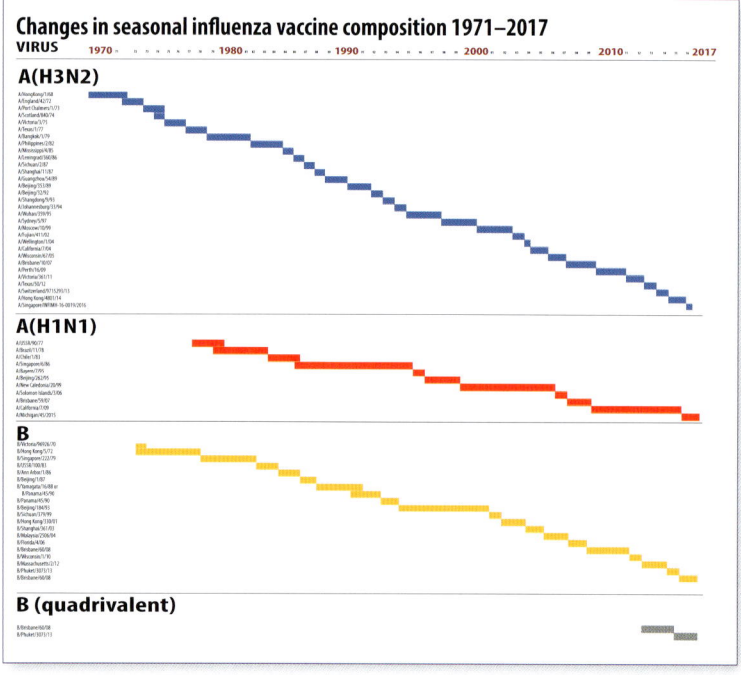

As of September 2017, WHO has recommended a total of 31 different H3N2 viruses, 11 H1N1 viruses and 20 influenza B viruses for use in seasonal influenza vaccines. Starting in 2012, recommendations for quadrivalent vaccines (which include both of the influenza B lineages) have also been issued.

During the first 25 years of GISRS, only a single seasonal influenza A subtype circulated in humans at any one time. However, in 1977 the two subtypes H3N2 and H1N1 began to co-circulate and seasonal vaccine recommendations therefore had to be made for both subtypes. Since 1972, 20 different influenza B vaccine viruses have also been recommended. Similarly, the complexity of making influenza B recommendations also increased when two distinct lineages of influenza B viruses (Victoria and Yamagata) began to co-circulate in the late 1980s. In September 2012, WHO began to make recommendations for both lineages of influenza B viruses to guide manufacturers wishing to produce a quadrivalent vaccine. As a result, current seasonal influenza vaccines are either trivalent or quadrivalent formulations, containing one influenza A H3N2 subtype, one influenza A H1N1 subtype, and either one or both influenza B viruses.

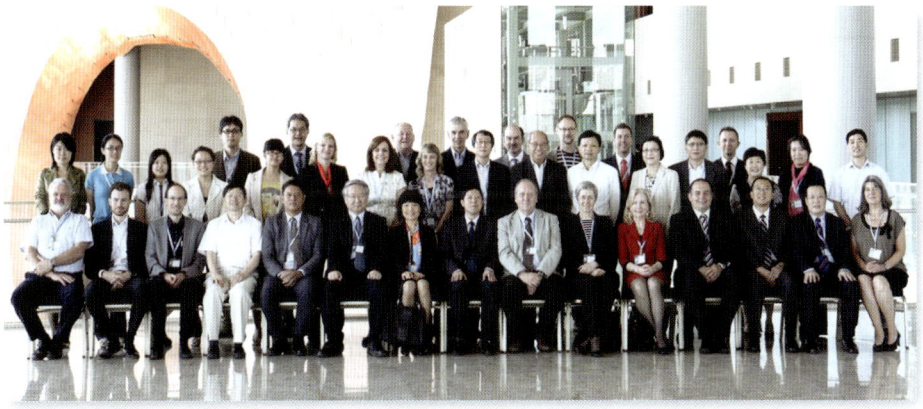

The WHO consultation on the composition of influenza virus vaccines for the southern hemisphere held in Beijing in 2012 was the first ever WHO vaccine composition meeting to make vaccine recommendations for both the Victoria and the Yamagata lineages of influenza B viruses.

In the lead-up to the biannual WHO vaccine composition meetings, experts from GISRS entities and other institutions hold regular teleconferences to efficiently exchange information. At the meeting itself, detailed and highly technical laboratory data are reviewed along with information on the epidemiological impact and geographical spread of variant viruses.

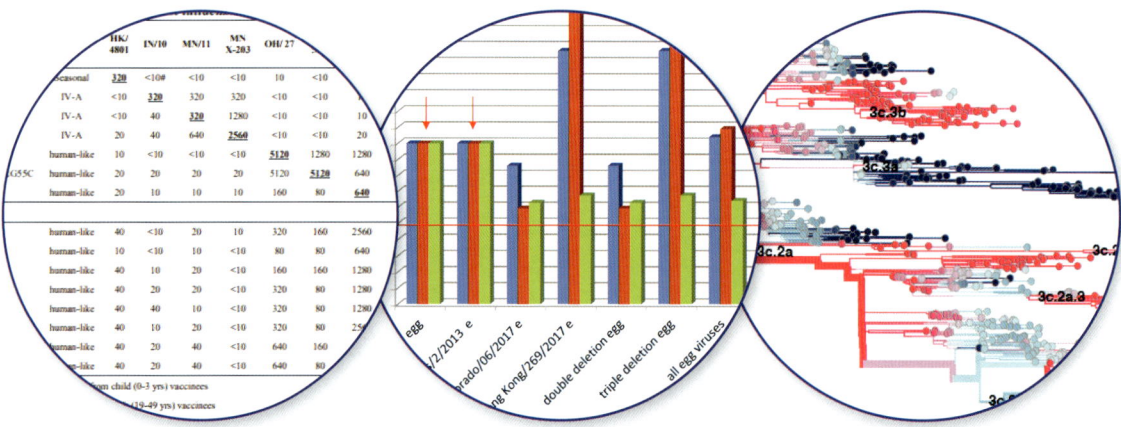

WHO seasonal influenza vaccine virus recommendations are based on expert review of highly complex datasets and other information generated by GISRS surveillance activities. Such data include (left to right) haemagglutinin inhibition titre tables, serological study results and phylogenetic "trees" showing the relatedness of different circulating viruses. Other important factors taken into account include the possible emergence of antiviral resistance, the results of vaccine-effectiveness studies and the availability of potential candidate vaccine viruses which grow well in eggs. In recent years, a number of potentially predictive mathematical modelling techniques have also been incorporated into the decision-making process.

Immediately after each vaccine composition meeting, the recommended composition of upcoming seasonal influenza vaccines is promptly communicated to vaccine manufacturers and the public, and the scientific basis for the decision is outlined. Many of the wild-type influenza viruses recommended for vaccine production grow very poorly in embryonated hens' eggs or cell cultures. If not addressed, such poor growth properties would significantly impact on vaccine production. WHOCCs therefore send the selected wild-type viruses to WHO ERLs and other specialized laboratories that use reassortment techniques in which the genetic material of two different influenza viruses are mixed to produce hybrid viruses suitable for vaccine production. The aim is to produce a virus containing the haemagglutinin and neuraminidase genes of the selected candidate vaccine virus along with the remaining gene segments of a virus with high growth properties.

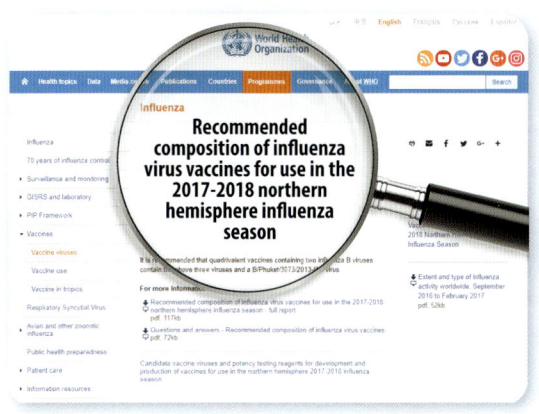

The properties of the resulting "high-growth reassortant" virus are then verified by genetic sequencing and antigenic characterization by WHOCCs. In addition, the virus is thoroughly tested for purity and stability, and its growth properties assessed, before it is made available to vaccine manufacturers.

During this time, WHO hosts regular teleconferences between vaccine manufacturers, WHOCCs and WHO ERLs in order to exchange views, provide updates on the progress made in developing high-growth reassortants and associated reagents, and share the results of yield evaluations carried out by manufacturers.

Upon receipt of the high-growth reassortant viruses, vaccine manufacturers carry out additional testing and then adapt the viruses to grow in their own growth substrate and culture conditions. Although the bulk of seasonal influenza vaccines are still prepared from viruses grown in embryonated hens' eggs – a technology dating back to the earliest days of vaccine production – several manufacturers are now also using cultured mammalian cell lines or recombinant DNA approaches to manufacture vaccines for human use.

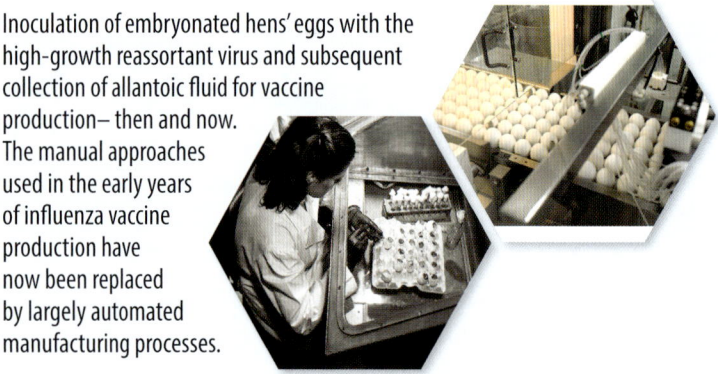

Inoculation of embryonated hens' eggs with the high-growth reassortant virus and subsequent collection of allantoic fluid for vaccine production – then and now. The manual approaches used in the early years of influenza vaccine production have now been replaced by largely automated manufacturing processes.

Because vaccine quality and potency need to be standardized and monitored as part of the regulatory and licensing process it is important that test reagents are produced by an independent and properly qualified source. WHO ERLs therefore produce these reagents and provide them to manufacturers – highlighting once again the key role played by GISRS laboratories throughout the entire course of vaccine development and production.

Once suitable viruses have been grown on a commercial scale, a number of different types of vaccines can be manufactured. Currently there are two types of seasonal influenza vaccines in clinical use – inactivated and live-attenuated vaccines. Inactivated vaccines contain intact influenza viruses (whole virus vaccines), viruses disrupted by detergent treatment (split virus vaccines), purified haemagglutinin and neuraminidase surface protein (subunit vaccines) or purified haemagglutinin obtained using recombinant technology. Viruses used for the production of live-attenuated vaccines are also prepared through reassortment but are grown in such a way that they cannot replicate at the temperatures typical of the human lower respiratory tract. This prevents the development of lower respiratory tract infections in individuals receiving the vaccine in the form of a nasal spray.

In the early years of seasonal influenza vaccination each vaccine dose was manually filled in reusable syringes under aseptic conditions immediately prior to injection.

With single-use syringes, the vaccination process today is far more efficient. This increased efficiency is a pre-requirement of successful mass vaccination campaigns.

The live-attenuated influenza vaccine is directly applied into the nostrils. This is less invasive than the intramuscular injection of inactivated vaccine.

The unique public–private partnership between GISRS and vaccine manufactures that drives the production of seasonal influenza vaccines stands as an exemplar of what can be achieved through close collaboration. Without this degree of collaboration, the production of such vaccines would simply not be possible. Under current technological constraints, seasonal vaccine production will always be a race against time, requiring a significant amount of scientifically informed and highly skilful prediction. This is a reality that very few outside the public health community are aware of. GISRS will continue to work with vaccine manufacturers and other partners to develop solutions, streamline processes and harness the exciting technological advances now emerging in this area.

By failing to prepare, you are preparing to fail.
                                          Benjamin Franklin

Preparing for the next pandemic
– constant vigilance and readiness to respond

Influenza pandemics have periodically swept through the human population for hundreds if not thousands of years. And what we know about the biology, epidemiology and ecology of influenza viruses leaves no doubt that another influenza pandemic is approaching. However, it is impossible to predict when this will occur and what impact it will have. Following concerted historical and epidemiological research in the 1990s a wealth of information on the impact of influenza pandemics during the twentieth century has now been gathered. This has led to the general and widely accepted understanding among the international influenza community and others that robust and sufficient preparations must be made well in advance if the world is to have any chance of promptly detecting and responding to a future pandemic.

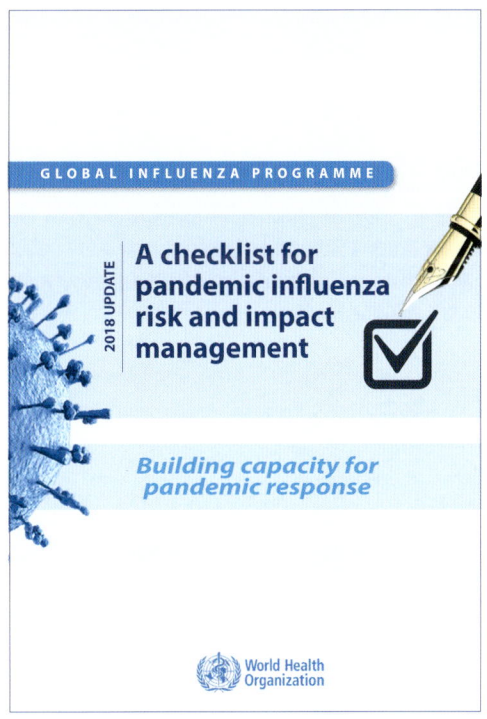

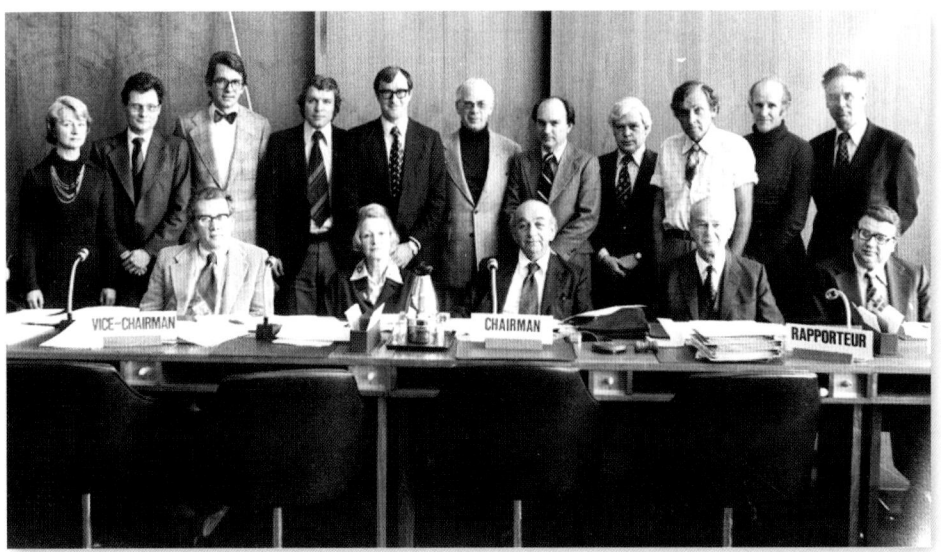

Long before the first cases of human H5N1 in Hong Kong SAR, China, in 1997 it was believed by some that animal influenza viruses presented an impending threat to public health. In the late 1970s, WHO held a Consultation on Influenza Ecology at which the animal reservoir for influenza viruses was discussed and potential threats identified.

It has also long been known that influenza is not the only respiratory pathogen capable of causing a devastating international health event. As the epidemics of SARS and MERS clearly demonstrated, major threats can also result from the spread of coronaviruses and other respiratory pathogens. In 1951, the Fourth World Health Assembly adopted the International Sanitary Regulations – a document developed to guide preparedness and response activities against international threats caused by infectious diseases. In 1969, the revised International Health Regulations (IHR) were adopted and then further amended in 1973 and 1981, with a focus placed primarily on yellow fever, plague and cholera.

Following the 2003 SARS outbreak – which caused over 8000 cases and almost 800 deaths across dozens of countries, the international community reviewed these earlier documents. In 2005, this resulted in the comprehensively revised IHR (2005) which is intended *to prevent, protect against, control and provide a public health response to the international spread of disease in ways that are commensurate with and restricted to public health risks, and which avoid unnecessary interference with international traffic and trade.*

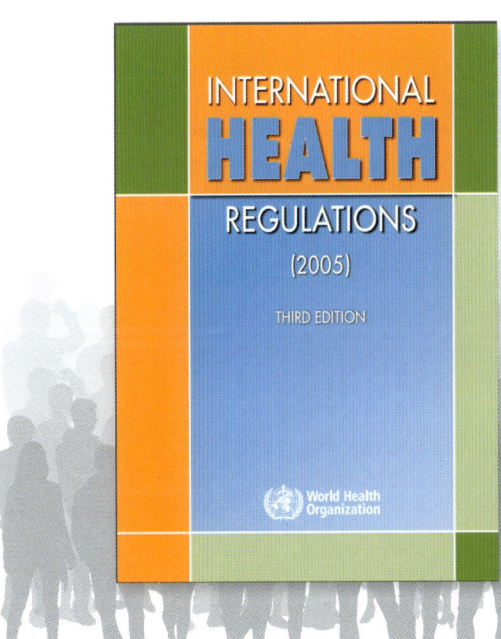

Member States have an obligation under IHR (2005) to report to WHO public health events that may constitute a public health emergency of international concern. The notification of such events takes into account certain criteria, such as the public health impact of the event, its risk of international spread, and the risk of travel or trade restrictions. Human influenza caused by a novel virus is one of the four diseases that must be reported immediately to WHO under IHR (2005) as this constitutes a serious and potentially rapidly evolving public health emergency.

Following the re-emergence of avian H5N1 influenza viruses causing human infections in 2003, numerous countries began to prepare or refine their national influenza pandemic preparedness plans. This prompted WHO to revise its existing guidance in this area – efforts in which GISRS played a central role. Previous WHO guidelines had outlined the actions to be taken by WHO and Member States during the different phases leading up to a pandemic, during the pandemic itself and during the scaling-down of actions as the world returned to an "interpandemic" phase. To better address the ongoing threat posed by H5N1 avian influenza viruses, updated guidelines had been produced in the lead-up to adoption of IHR (2005). The adoption of the new regulations then prompted a wealth of new research and expert views on how best to prepare for an influenza pandemic – along with advances such as the international stockpiling of antiviral drugs. In 2009, WHO produced corresponding guidance in accordance with these and other developments. This guidance reflected the knowledge and experience gained in dealing with severe pandemics, such as the 1918 Spanish flu pandemic, and with the potentially catastrophic threats posed by animal influenza viruses such as H5N1.

The subsequent advent of the far less disruptive 2009 H1N1 influenza pandemic, and the lessons learnt in responding to it, sharply highlighted the need for preparedness approaches capable of more flexibly dealing with a whole range of potential threats of differing severity. This signalled a shift away from the phase-based approaches taken in previous WHO guidelines and towards a risk-based approach in which Member States were encouraged to develop flexible influenza pandemic preparedness plans. This approach requires national assessments of the actual risk posed during any emerging event, taking into account the global risk assessments conducted by WHO which are based in large part on the virological and other information generated by GISRS.

The lessons learnt during the 2009 H1N1 pandemic led to a fundamental shift towards a far more flexible national risk-based approach...

As part of this shift towards a risk-based approach, the development of new WHO guidelines informed by GISRS expertise was undertaken, with a far stronger emphasis placed on the conducting and applying of risk and severity assessments. This culminated in 2017 in the publication of the WHO document *Pandemic influenza risk management*. One key development in this document is its enhanced alignment with existing national and United Nations policies and approaches for managing the risk of any natural or man-made disaster in the broader context of an "all hazards" approach. Such an approach accords very naturally with the long-established emphasis placed by GISRS on the crucial importance of national capacity-building and associated preparedness efforts as the foundation of response and recovery activities.

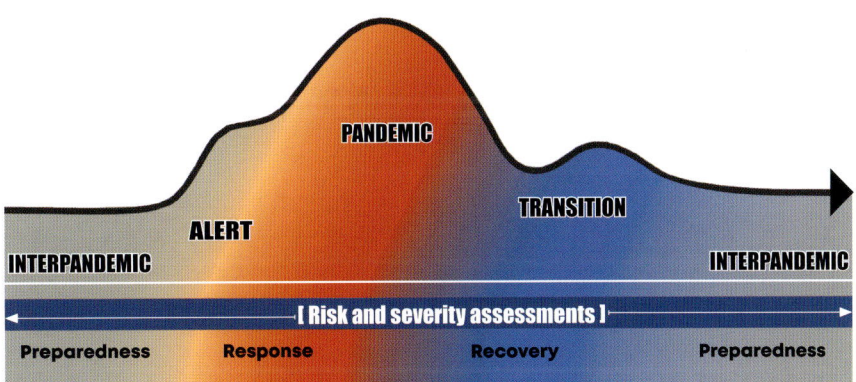

Based on the most up-to-date virological, epidemiological and clinical knowledge, and informed by the long history of GISRS activities, current WHO guidance greatly simplifies the global phases of a pandemic. These global phases have now been uncoupled from risk-management decisions and actions at the country level, with Member States encouraged to use national risk assessments based on their specific situation and needs to guide decision-making.

TIPRA was developed to provide a standardized and transparent approach for assessing the risk of a pandemic caused by a particular influenza virus strain.

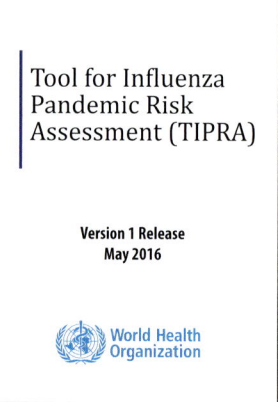

Given the continuous threat to global public health posed by influenza viruses with pandemic potential, WHO has also prepared the *Tool for Influenza Pandemic Risk Assessment (TIPRA)*. TIPRA was developed to provide a standardized and transparent approach for assessing the risk of a pandemic caused by a particular influenza virus strain. In the event of an outbreak, GISRS experts will evaluate the likelihood of the virus spreading through human-to-human transmission and the likely public health impact this would have. As part of this process, TIPRA will be used to systematically identify any gaps in the knowledge and information required to make an informed judgement.

Once TIPRA has been used to assess the level of hazard associated with a specific virus, each country can then take into consideration their national context and likely levels of exposure. The result of this systematic three-part analysis would then be used to guide the risk-management actions appropriate to each country.

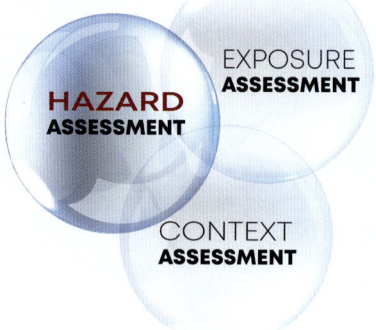

Year-round seasonal influenza vaccine production, distribution and timely administration is the bedrock of pandemic vaccine production and rapid deployment.

Once the start of the next influenza pandemic has been announced, the ability of countries and the global health community to respond will rely upon already established and well-functioning seasonal influenza activities and capacities. Nowhere is this reliance more apparent than in the area of vaccine availability during a pandemic. Year-round seasonal influenza vaccine production, distribution and timely administration is the bedrock of pandemic vaccine production and rapid deployment – without such pre-existing capacities and processes no pandemic influenza vaccine could possibly be manufactured in sufficient quantity or deployed quickly enough to those in most need during an emergency. In addition, production facilities cannot be used to produce seasonal and pandemic vaccines at the same time. This unavoidably means that supplies of seasonal influenza vaccine would be drastically affected, with potentially serious public health consequences in its own right.

GISRS will continue to work to ensure the prompt detection of any emerging pandemic influenza threat, monitor the unfolding situation, and collect and share viruses and related information. GISRS will also continue to be centrally involved in informal consultations and other meetings aimed at strengthening the pandemic preparedness of countries in key areas such as deciding upon the exact point at which seasonal influenza vaccine production should be switched to pandemic vaccine production.

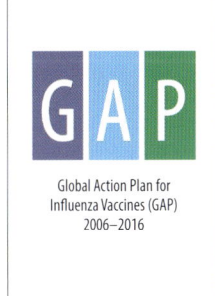

Global Action Plan for Influenza Vaccines (GAP) 2006–2016

Global Action Plan for Influenza Vaccines (GAP) 2006–2016 was a comprehensive strategy which aimed to address the global shortage of influenza vaccines for use in both seasonal epidemics and pandemics by: (a) increasing seasonal influenza vaccine use; (b) increasing influenza vaccine production capacity; and (c) accelerating vaccine research and the development of more effective vaccines.

Adoption of the PIP Framework in May 2011 – a landmark event in international public health.

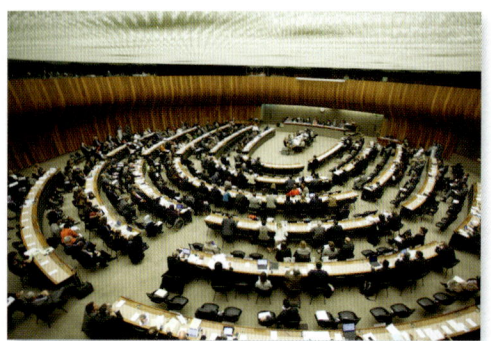

Following the re-emergence of human cases of infection with avian H5N1 viruses in 2003 and the subsequent rapid spread of these viruses among domesticated birds in several Asian countries , it became clear to WHO Member States that a formal arrangement was needed to increase access to pandemic vaccines by countries in need. Member States also recognized the crucial need for rapid and systematic virus sharing to ensure continuous global monitoring and risk assessment, and the development of safe and effective pandemic vaccines.

In 2007, Member States began formal and informal discussions, interacting with industry, civil society organizations and other stakeholders, to develop the PIP Framework. After its unanimous adoption by the Sixty-fourth World Health Assembly on 24 May 2011, the PIP Framework was hailed as a landmark achievement in bringing together both the public and private sectors in an unprecedented partnership for global public health.

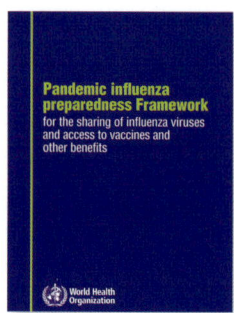

With GISRS firmly at the centre of global pandemic preparedness and response activities, the PIP Framework identifies specific responsibilities for both WHO Member States and other stakeholders. For their part, Member States are expected to support their NICs and to ensure the rapid, systematic and timely sharing of influenza viruses with pandemic potential with GISRS WHOCCs to allow for comprehensive risk assessment and the development of candidate pandemic vaccine viruses for use by industry.

In turn, manufacturers of influenza vaccines, pharmaceuticals or diagnostics must pay an annual Partnership Contribution to WHO if they use GISRS. WHO uses the Partnership Contribution funds to strengthen preparedness capacities – including surveillance and laboratory skills – in countries where they are weak. WHO also works to strengthen national regulatory agencies to facilitate the prompt approval and deployment of pandemic vaccines and medicines provided during a pandemic. The Partnership Contribution also allows WHO to build up a reserve of funds that can be used as soon as a pandemic virus emerges so that critical response activities can be rapidly implemented. Manufacturers must also sign a legally binding "Standard Material Transfer Agreement-2" (SMTA2) when receiving PIP biological materials from GISRS. In this way, WHO can secure predictable and timely access to life-saving vaccines, antivirals and other supplies needed during a pandemic. By putting these agreements in place now, WHO, its Member States and industry are all working together to ensure that when the next pandemic starts the access to critical life-saving supplies by all countries will be fairer and more efficient.

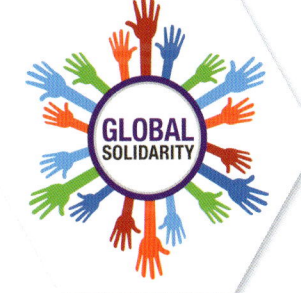

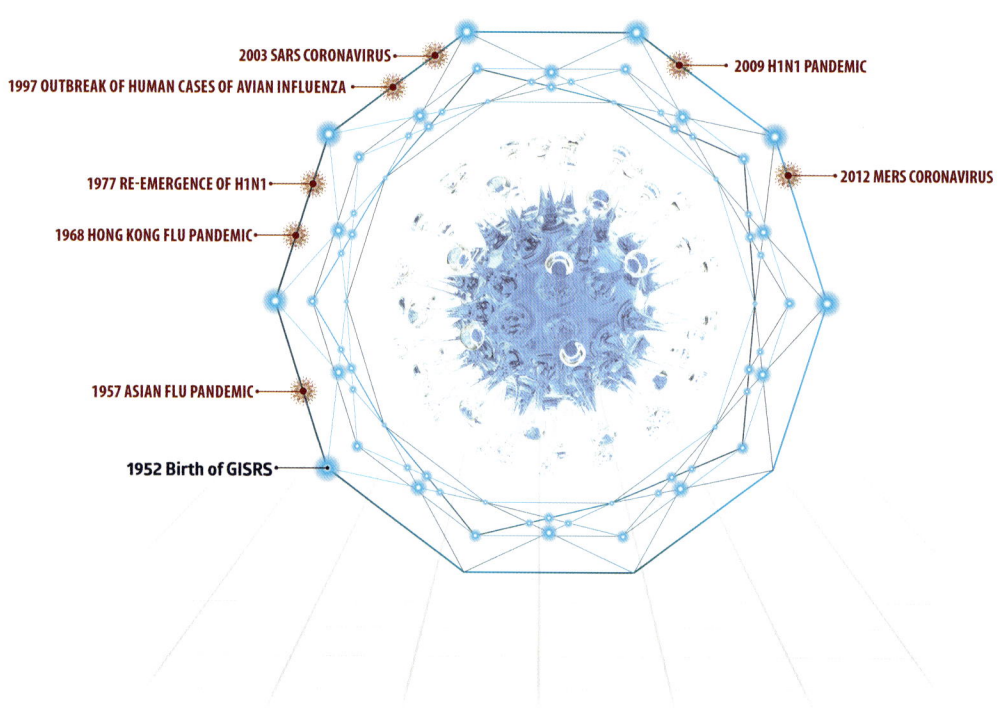

A long history of responding to emergencies

Since its establishment in 1952, GISRS has rapidly and comprehensively responded to a series of highly challenging public health emergencies. These have included three influenza pandemics, numerous cases of human infection with animal influenza viruses such as H5N1 and H7N9, and two potentially devastating coronavirus outbreaks.

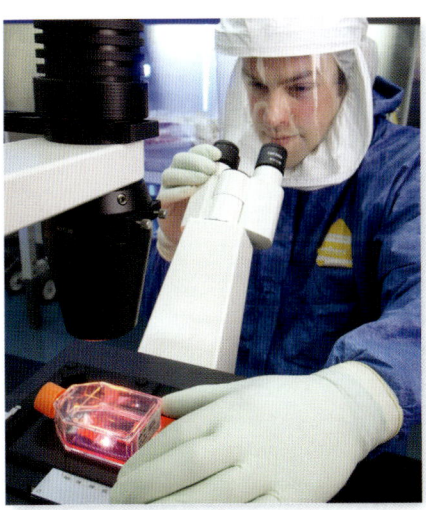
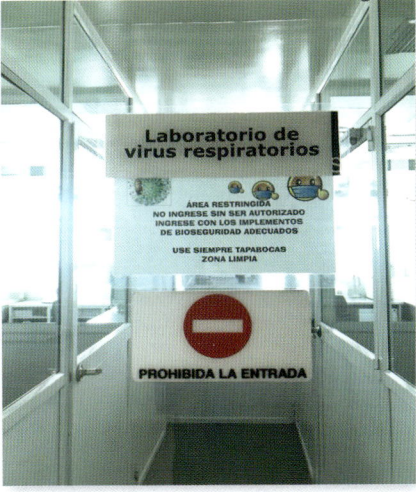

On 4 May 1957 – only 5 years after the establishment of GISRS – WHO was informed by the Singapore NIC that an influenza A virus had been isolated that was antigenically distinct from the then circulating seasonal H1N1 subtype. This notification signalled the beginning of the "Asian flu" pandemic caused by the H2N2 subtype. The virus was quickly characterized by the World Influenza Centre in London and by the Walter Reed Army Institute for Research in Washington, DC. GISRS responded swiftly by distributing freeze-dried virus samples to all 57 NICs in 46 countries to enable them to prepare appropriate diagnostic reagents – a crucial step in surveillance and response efforts. A WHO statement issued at the time remains as true today as it was then:

> *What the network of WHO influenza centres offers every country is the fruit of a carefully coordinated international collaboration, that is prompt identification of the virus, detection of epidemics in their early stages, early warnings to health authorities of impending danger, dispatch of freeze-dried virus samples, specialist advice and assistance in the training of technicians. These are the means which are now being employed in an attempt to limit the effects of pandemic influenza.*

Eleven years later, in 1968, the "Hong Kong flu" pandemic caused by the influenza H3N2 subtype swept across the world, affecting all age groups. Studies at the World Influenza Centre and elsewhere quickly indicated that the previously used H2N2 vaccine would not provide a sufficient level of protection against this new virus subtype. As the pandemic progressed, surveillance by GISRS laboratories revealed important global and regional variations in patterns of illness and death. In Japan and Western Europe, for example, the initial epidemics tended to be small, scattered and very mild – only becoming much more severe and deadly the following year. This stood in sharp contrast to the high rates of illness and death in the USA immediately following the introduction of the virus on the West Coast.

Among the insights made possible by these GISRS monitoring and response efforts was the realization that under certain circumstances the second wave of a pandemic has the potential to be worse than the initial wave. As the twentieth century progressed, the sheer unpredictability of influenza outbreaks and the complex considerations that needed to be taken into account to ensure rapid responses to real threats while avoiding over-reactions to others become more and more apparent with each event. Even today, predicting the complex dynamics and likely severity of an influenza pandemic remains hugely challenging.

In 1976, a classical H1N1 swine influenza virus caused illness among conscripts and other military personnel at the Fort Dix army training centre in New Jersey, USA. In accordance with the scientific understanding of the day it was concluded by some influenza experts that this was likely to be the start of a new H1N1 pandemic and rapid response activities were undertaken, including the partial roll-out of a national vaccination programme in the USA. However, the event proved self-limiting and today this and subsequent similar events are viewed as transient clusters of human infections with zoonotic influenza viruses that require continual monitoring by GISRS and other laboratories to ensure that the countermeasures taken are both prompt and proportionate.

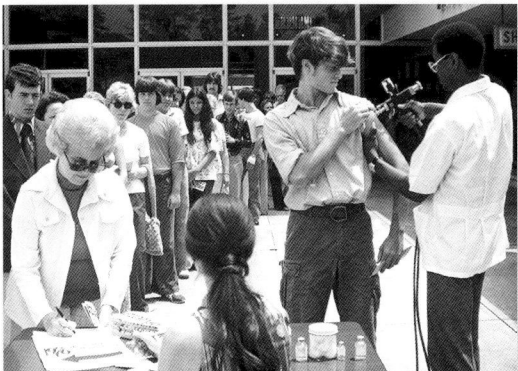

The threat of a pandemic leaves no room for complacency.

What is known for certain is that the threat of a pandemic leaves no room for complacency. On 24 April 2009, the WHOCC, Atlanta informed WHO of two cases of influenza in two unrelated children in southern California caused by an H1N1 virus of swine origin. These cases had been preceded by outbreaks of influenza-like infections in Mexico – some of which had been very severe. Almost immediately GISRS was able to confirm the causative virus strain and the Director-General of WHO announced a "Public Health Emergency of International Concern" that was to become the 2009 H1N1 pandemic. This event would once again push GISRS to the frontline of global human health.

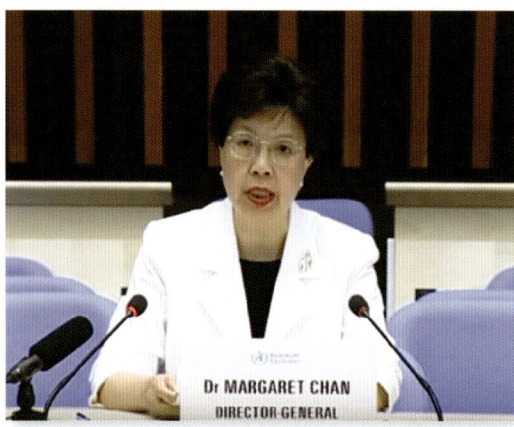

On 11 June 2009, the Director-General of WHO, Dr Margaret Chan, declared the start of the 2009 H1N1 influenza pandemic in the Executive Board Room at WHO headquarters. This announcement signalled the first influenza pandemic of the new millennium.

Almost immediately after the announcement, the genetic data needed to develop vital molecular diagnostics were uploaded by GISRS to publically accessible genetic sequence databases. Within 7 days of receiving clinical specimens, the WHOCC in Atlanta had developed diagnostic protocols and kits which were then provided to NICs and other laboratories worldwide. During 2009, NICs used these kits to test more than two million clinical specimens and reported the results weekly to WHO.

Within 31 days of the identification and full characterization of the causative virus by GISRS laboratories – and evaluation of the risk it presented – WHO issued recommendations for the A/California/7/2009 vaccine virus to be used in a pandemic vaccine. One day later this was followed by the provision of a high-growth candidate vaccine virus by GISRS laboratories to vaccine manufacturers. It is no exaggeration to say that the 2009 H1N1 pandemic helped forge GISRS into the resilient and flexible global health resource it is today. Without the expertise, professionalism and collaborative spirit of GISRS internal and external partners, and the coordinating of crucial resources and activities, it is difficult to envisage how the world could have ever responded so swiftly to such a rapidly emerging threat.

Following the pandemic, the Director-General of WHO proposed that an IHR Review Committee be convened to review the experience gained and lessons learnt during the pandemic. After extensive and lengthy deliberations the Review Committee concluded that GISRS had:

> ...*facilitated rapid sharing and analysis of virological specimens throughout the pandemic ... [and] had worked well and facilitated the timely detection, identification, initial characterization and monitoring of the pandemic (H1N1) 2009 virus ... the first time that a worldwide laboratory initiative was well-coordinated for an extended period of time.*

Human cases of infection with an animal influenza virus were a wake-up call that any novel influenza virus might make the leap to humans and cause the next influenza pandemic.

In 1997, the belief that differences in virus receptors in birds and humans would prevent human infection with highly pathogenic avian influenza viruses such as H5N1 ("bird flu") was shown to be dangerously incorrect. Of the 18 individuals infected that year through contact with infected poultry in Hong Kong SAR, China, six died – underlining the deadly nature of such "zoonotic" infections. On this occasion the depopulation of live bird markets proved to be an effective strategy for stopping the outbreak as no human-to-human transmission had yet occurred. However, the occurrence of human cases of infection with an animal influenza virus was a wake-up call that any such viruses, of whatever subtype, might at any moment make the leap to humans and cause the next influenza pandemic.

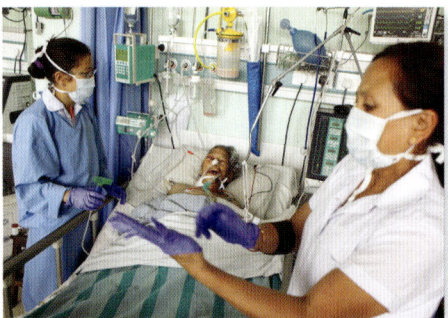
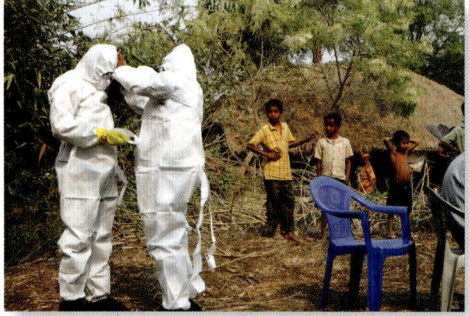

Since the 1997 H5N1 outbreak a number of avian influenza virus subtypes have caused numerous zoonotic infections. These infections are often severe, require intensive hospital care and are associated with very high case-fatality rates. In addition, because H5N1 viruses also cause devastating animal outbreaks in poultry farms and backyard flocks, infected and uninfected animals need to be destroyed. This directly results in substantial and often catastrophic economic losses for farmers and the poultry industry.

In recent years, sporadic human cases of influenza caused by avian H7N9 viruses have also highlighted the importance of rapid detection and response in relation to an emerging threat. Until March 2013, this particular virus had not been observed in either animals or people. By 10 April, WHOCCs and WHO ERLs had received viruses, and within a month the first candidate vaccine virus was developed. As quickly as 31 May 2013, WHO was able to issue recommendations on the development of H7N9 vaccines. Since that time WHO has provided regular and frequent situation updates on the occurrence of human infections with H7N9 and other avian influenza viruses on the WHO website, and has provided updated recommendations for candidate vaccine virus development as necessary.

Animal influenza viruses capable of causing human infections thus present a significant public health challenge. Because in each case the virus reservoir occurs in animals such as domestic poultry and pigs, effective collaboration between GISRS and the animal health sector is crucial. Since 2004, a number of joint initiatives have been undertaken between GISRS and veterinary laboratories, and in 2005 the OIE–FAO[1] Network of Expertise on Animal Influenza (OFFLU) was established to coordinate the global surveillance of animal influenza. If the public health sector is to meet the challenges to health posed by H5N1, H7N9 and other animal influenza viruses such collaboration will increasingly be crucial.

[1] World Organisation for Animal Health–Food and Agriculture Organization of the United Nations.

And nor is influenza the only respiratory virus threat facing the world.

And nor is influenza the only respiratory virus threat facing the world. In 2003, a mysterious pathogen causing severe and often fatal respiratory infections emerged in Asia. As the unidentified pathogen spread and the level of global concern rapidly escalated, GISRS and other scientists worked to rapidly identify the zoonotic coronavirus responsible for SARS. Following its initial transmission from civet cats to humans the SARS coronavirus acquired the capacity for human-to-human transmission. Between the beginning of November 2002 and the end of July 2003, a total of 8096 human cases had been reported to WHO across 32 countries with 774 fatalities.

The severity of SARS symptoms, its apparent ease of spread and the rapid appearance of cases among health care workers led WHO to issue a global alert in March 2003. This contributed to the implementation of personal hygiene and other protection measures which were instrumental in halting its spread. In July 2003 WHO declared that the outbreak had been stopped.

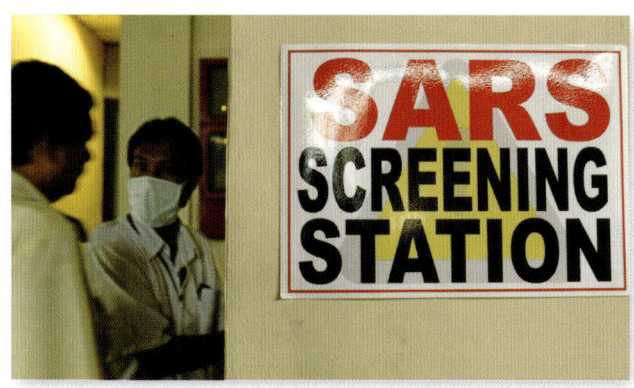

GISRS has long been at the forefront of the world's defences against infectious respiratory viruses.

Starting in September 2012, GISRS laboratories have also been centrally involved in the response to the threat posed by the MERS coronavirus – another zoonotic coronavirus, this time believed to have first been transmitted to humans from infected camels. By the end of 2017, WHO had been notified of 2122 laboratory-confirmed human cases of infection with the MERS coronavirus in 27 countries, resulting in 740 deaths.

Whether faced with a potential influenza pandemic, outbreaks of zoonotic infection or disease outbreaks caused by respiratory viruses other than influenza, GISRS has over its long history repeatedly demonstrated its capacity to rapidly detect and respond to emergency situations. With its global reach, collaborative ethos and risk-based approach, GISRS has long been at the forefront of the world's defences against infectious respiratory viruses.

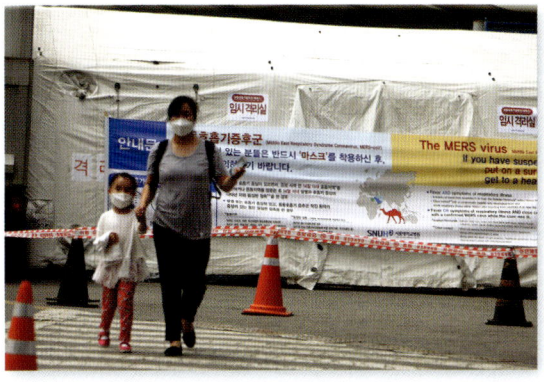

The MERS coronavirus remains a very real threat today – here a mother and daughter in the Republic of Korea wear face masks in front of a health advisory sign at a quarantine tent for potentially infected people.

*Nothing in life is to be feared, it is only to be understood.
Now is the time to understand more, so that we may fear less.*
                                                    Marie Curie

Harnessing technology and furthering knowledge

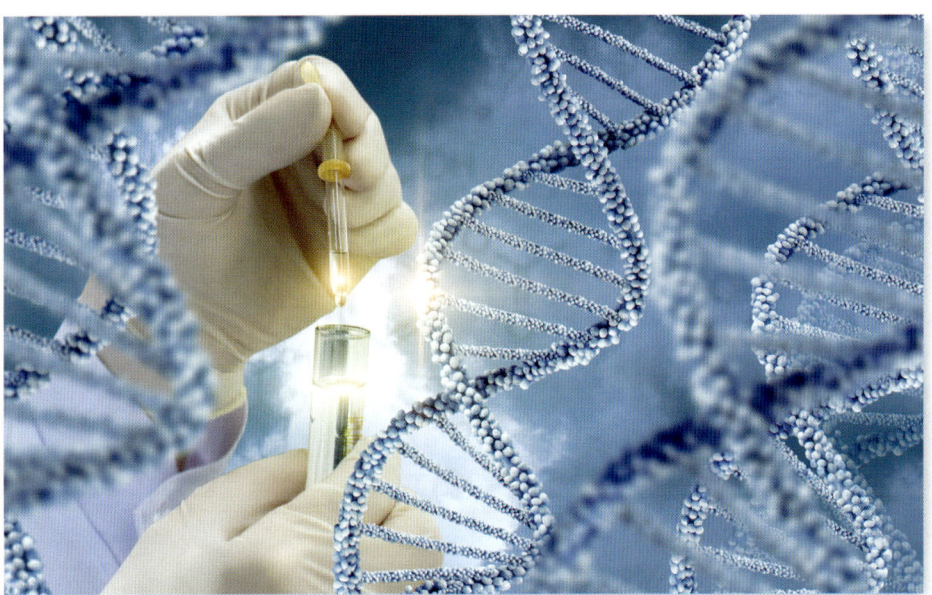

When GISRS was established in 1952 there were only a few laboratory techniques available for diagnosing influenza and characterizing the causative virus. These techniques were essentially limited to culturing viruses in embryonated hens' eggs or in monkey kidney cell cultures and then subjecting them to further analysis using complement-fixation, haemagglutination-inhibition and neutralization assays. Although these methods continue to be used for GISRS laboratory investigations and vaccine virus recommendations, recent decades have seen dramatic technological developments and advances in knowledge. Today, GISRS is increasingly adopting and refining a wide range of technologies, many of which lie at the cutting edge of current understanding of virus evolution and vaccine development.

Despite continual refinement of these traditional methods and approaches, there have always been problems and limitations associated with their use. In recent years, a number of fundamental technical issues have arisen leading to significant difficulties in detecting and accurately characterizing circulating influenza viruses, particularly H3N2 viruses. GISRS laboratories have responded to these technical challenges by implementing a wide range of innovative solutions and sharing the insights gained.

In 1931 the discovery that influenza viruses could be grown in large numbers in embryonated hens' eggs was a breakthrough in influenza research. It not only allowed for the use of relatively rapid and sensitive diagnostic and virus characterization techniques but also opened the way to the safe production of influenza vaccines. Today, the procedure continues to be a vital step in the detailed laboratory characterization of viruses and is still the main method used to produce vaccines on an industrial scale.

In the 1940s cell culture techniques were developed for the propagation of many different viruses, including influenza viruses. Despite a gap of several decades and significant improvements in technique, many of the underlying principles remain the same, with both virologists shown here using an inverted microscope to examine cell cultures for the characteristic microscopic changes caused by influenza viruses.

For example, since the 1940s the antigenic characterization of influenza viruses has been based on their natural ability to cause red blood cells to tightly clump together (a process known as "haemagglutination"). The degree to which this clumping together is prevented by the presence of antibodies is the basis of the haemagglutination inhibition assay. Even today, this historic assay lies at the heart of the GISRS vaccine virus selection and development process. In recent years however, the seasonal H3N2 influenza viruses have progressively displayed a reduced tendency to haemagglutinate red blood cells from a range of animal species. GISRS laboratories have responded to this and related challenges by refining the current procedure, working to improve the standardization of newer laboratory methods, and supporting research into the development of currently experimental but highly promising technological advances such as the use of synthetic red blood cells and the production of panels of recombinant haemagglutinin proteins.

Another issue currently requiring attention is the poor growth of influenza H3N2 viruses in both embryonated eggs and commonly used cell lines. Successful solutions developed by GISRS laboratories to the increasingly poor growth of H3N2 viruses in eggs have included the use of eggs from a specific breed of hen, increasing the age at which embryonated eggs are inoculated, changing the inoculation route to the allantoic cavity and increasing the incubation temperature from 33 °C to 35 °C.

To add to the complexity, H3N2 viruses can also exhibit unwanted genetic adaptations caused by the substrate (egg or cell culture) that they are grown in. Although such adaptations promote high levels of growth they can also make the affected viruses antigenically distinct from the wild-type circulating virus. When tested using conventional laboratory assays, egg-grown and cell-grown viruses can then exhibit different reactions to the exact same antibody, thus complicating analysis of their antigenic properties. This is particularly true for viruses grown in eggs, and so GISRS laboratories routinely use viruses grown in each substrate during virus characterization to reveal precisely how the substrate used affects their antigenic properties.

The widespread application of so-called "molecular methods" in the 1990s signalled the start of a new era in the fight against infectious diseases.

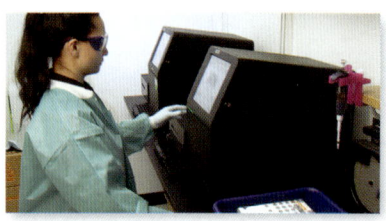

The widespread application of so-called "molecular methods" for identifying viruses and other pathogens in the 1990s signalled the start of a new era in the fight against influenza. For the first time, the haemagglutinin, neuraminidase and other virus genes of interest could be sequenced to enable the rapid and highly accurate detection of influenza viruses using nucleic acid amplification-based techniques, such as the reverse-transcription polymerase chain reaction (RT-PCR). Since its initial application in detecting seasonal influenza viruses in humans the use of RT-PCR has been expanded to detect H5N1, H7N9 and other zoonotic influenza virus subtypes, as well as Yamagata and Victoria lineages of influenza B viruses. The assay is now the primary method used in NICs and other laboratories to detect influenza viruses in clinical specimens, and produces highly sensitive and specific results within hours.

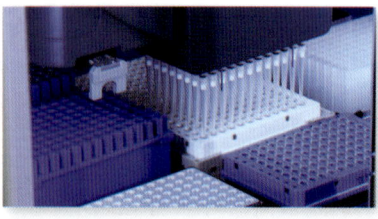

Today, next-generation genetic sequencing technologies also allow for entire virus genomes, not just individual genes, to be very rapidly sequenced. Such technologies have the potential to bring about a revolution in influenza surveillance, associated risk assessment and the selection and development of candidate vaccine viruses. Combining the data obtained from genetic sequencing with the results of more traditional laboratory assays can already provide timely and crucial information on the evolution, virulence and likely antiviral susceptibility of circulating influenza viruses. One clear challenge at present is finding ways of matching the enormous volumes of data generated with corresponding capacities for data management, analysis, understanding and dissemination.

Other emerging techniques include the use of antigenic cartography which elegantly combines the results of traditional haemagglutination inhibition tests with genetic sequence data and visualizes the results over time. Although this technique has for over a decade made an important contribution to the biannual WHO vaccine composition meetings, the full range of its potential application in areas such as the complex patterns of protection conferred by prior immunity is still being evaluated.

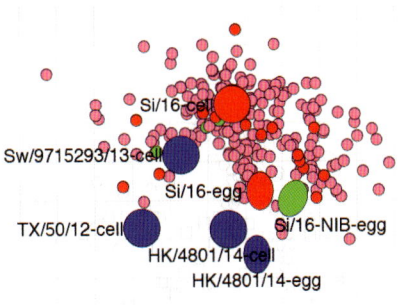

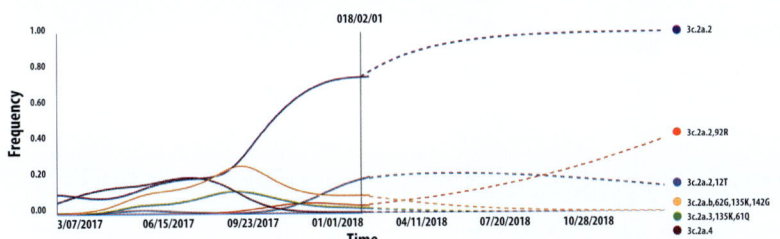

A number of potentially predictive mathematical modelling approaches have also been developed in recent years and their practical application in the GISRS vaccine virus selection process is now being explored.

Next-generation genetic sequencing on an industrial scale, antigenic cartography and mathematical modelling are among the many approaches currently being evaluated for their utility in monitoring, characterizing and predicting the evolution of influenza viruses, and are increasingly being incorporated into the activities of GISRS. As the pace of scientific innovation accelerates, these exciting and potentially revolutionary advances are bringing the prospect of entirely new ways of understanding the origin and course of both seasonal epidemics and potential pandemics, and of rapidly producing well-matched vaccines.

The advent of the World Wide Web changed the face of data collection and information sharing forever.

It is not only in the laboratory that GISRS looks to improve its functioning and expand its reach. Comprehensive influenza surveillance also relies upon the timely exchange of related epidemiological and virological information. In the decades since 1952, GISRS communications approaches have undergone a remarkable transformation. During the earliest years, the WHO *Weekly Epidemiological Record*, regular mail and the telephone were the primary means of communication. Although the invention of telex and telefax accelerated the exchange of information, it was the digital communications revolution which truly transformed this area.

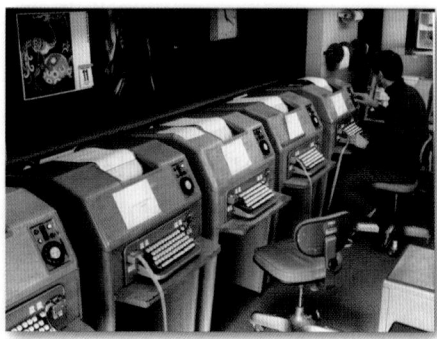

Early communications technologies such as the telex room in WHO headquarters have now given way to the almost instantaneous uploading of data from laboratories all round the world to the WHO FluNet database.

The advent of the World Wide Web changed the face of data collection and information sharing forever. In collaboration with the Institut National de la Santé et de la Recherche Médicale, WHO developed the internet-based "FluNet" data-collection and reporting tool. By using this online resource NICs and WHOCCs can now instantly share information in real time with other GISRS laboratories, WHO and the public. The WHO Global Influenza Programme also maintains a discussion forum and information-exchange platform which is used for the rapid exchange of information between GISRS laboratories.

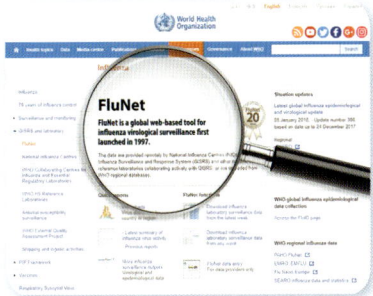

As more and more countries have developed influenza virus genome sequencing capacity, several publically accessible databases for uploading influenza virus genetic sequence data and related information have been established. These include the Global Initiative on Sharing All Influenza Data (GISAID) EpiFlu database, which in a spirit of openness promotes the international sharing of influenza virus sequences, related human clinical and epidemiological data, and information on avian and other animal viruses. In the USA the GenBank genetic sequence database is part of the International Nucleotide Sequence Database Collaboration (INSDC) which also contains databases and archives from Europe and Japan. Both the GISAID and INSDC databases and related resources are regularly consulted by GISRS laboratories and other partners.

It is now clear that a number of new technologies and associated tools have the potential to revolutionize traditional influenza surveillance, and associated risk assessment and response activities. Alongside this, further scientific understanding of the complex biology and ecology of influenza viruses will also be needed. Given long-standing shortfalls in national, regional and global influenza surveillance and response capacities, it has long been recognized that simply maintaining the status quo will not be enough. As laboratory assays, genetic sequencing, information-sharing, mathematical-modelling and other technologies continue to evolve GISRS will continue to play its full part in driving forward their development and adoption.

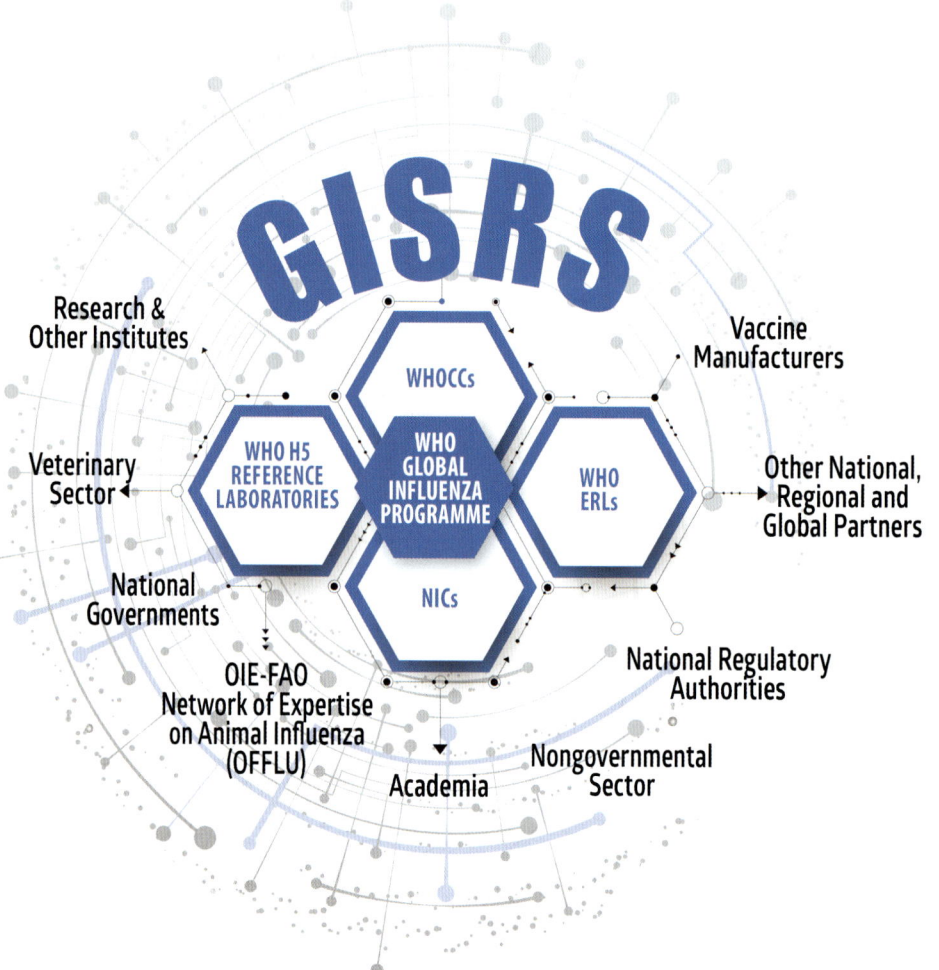

Working together
– the driving force of GISRS

The history of GISRS stands as an exemplar of how a wide range of key stakeholders working together can make a huge contribution to global public health and health security. Not only has GISRS learnt from other networks conducting infectious disease surveillance and response activities but it has in return served as a model for other networks, new and old. It is the continuing close collaboration between GISRS member institutes and numerous external partners and stakeholders that makes possible the delivery of a wide range of public health and health security benefits. These include the streamlined and timely exchange of viruses and related information, the worldwide provision of reagents and laboratory protocols, the timely development and production of vaccines, strengthened seasonal and pandemic preparedness and response activities and capacities, and provision of invaluable training opportunities. In addition, scientists working within GISRS have not only developed new methods but have also adopted cutting-edge technologies developed elsewhere.

When faced with such a rapidly evolving threat as influenza, such collaboration is crucial. Seasonal influenza viruses tend to spread very rapidly through the first-affected communities, typically causing epidemics which last weeks and months, with their wider spread to other areas occurring in the weeks and months which follow. Influenza viruses with pandemic potential could potentially spread from one continent to another in a matter of hours and then go on to encircle the entire globe within weeks. Without the commitment and collaboration demonstrated year after year by GISRS and all its partners, none of the public health and health security gains described in this book would be possible.

Collaboration between WHOCCs, NICs and WHO ERLs takes place continuously throughout the year...

It is NICs and other national laboratories participating in influenza surveillance that contribute the most precious materials, namely the influenza viruses circulating in their respective countries, along with information on their epidemiological impact. WHOCCs are in regular contact with NICs and routinely provide them with expert advice and support in their day-to-day influenza surveillance activities. To strengthen NIC capacities WHOCCs and other GISRS laboratories also provide frequent training courses and other learning opportunities to NIC staff in order to increase their proficiency in specific laboratory methods, and to familiarize staff from different laboratories in the use of state-of-the-art techniques. In many cases, the detailed instructions, laboratory protocols and background information provided in the course materials are translated into the language(s) of the country or region where the courses are being held.

In addition to holding external training courses for smaller and larger groups, WHOCCs and other GISRS laboratories also invite virologists from all over the world to be trained in-house in specific methods. This not only helps to build national laboratory capacities and introduce new technological developments but also strengthens the strong collegial ethos at the heart of GISRS.

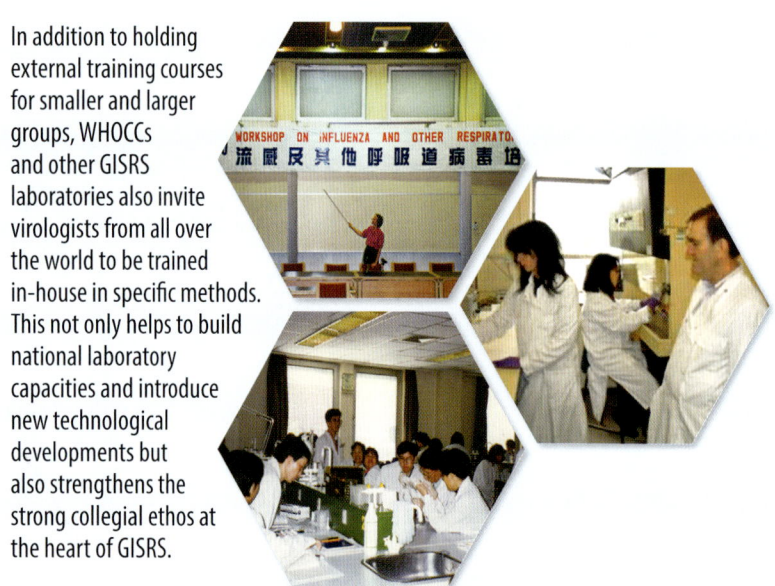

For decades, WHOCCs, NICs and WHO ERLs have been key drivers of much of the scientific and methodological progress made in the field of influenza. Often operating with only limited resources, these GISRS entities have made great strides in furthering scientific understanding of the nature of influenza viruses and their evolution. Collaboration between WHOCCs, NICs and WHO ERLs takes place continuously throughout the year, and between them these institutions take on the bulk of the work leading to the biannual WHO recommendations on candidate vaccine viruses. This work ranges from the antigenic analysis and genetic sequencing of viruses, antiviral sensitivity testing, human serology studies and the preparation of influenza reagent kits. WHOCCs and WHO ERLs then collaborate closely in the preparation of candidate vaccine viruses and the development of high-growth reassortant strains.

For many years, the Centers for Disease Control and Prevention, through its Influenza Division and associated WHOCC, Atlanta, has provided considerable technical, logistical and financial support for GISRS activities. This includes the free provision each year of a reagent kit to all NICs worldwide. This kit contains the sera, monoclonal antibodies and antigens needed to characterize circulating influenza viruses.

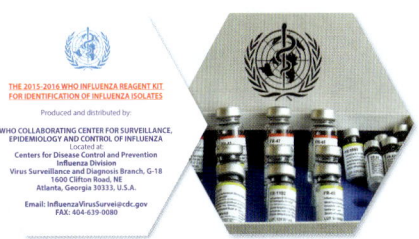

The re-emergence of avian H5N1 influenza viruses causing zoonotic infections in 2003 resulted in a number of laboratories becoming designated as WHO H5 Reference Laboratories and becoming a key part of GISRS. These specialized laboratories have frequently demonstrated their ability to rapidly identify and characterize unusual subtypes of influenza viruses. Such laboratories were able to rapidly provide support to countries which did not have the capacity to safely handle such viruses at the time of their emergence. Since then, there have been significant capacity-building gains made in many countries with the required laboratory biosafety levels and other requirements now in place as part of routine NIC activities.

Through the years, WHO manuals have been an invaluable tool for NICs in diagnosing infection and characterizing viruses in accordance with the highest available standards. In 1982, WHO produced a laboratory manual which for almost 30 years set out in detail the methods to be used for the detection and characterization of influenza viruses. In 2011, this manual was extensively revised and expanded by GISRS experts.

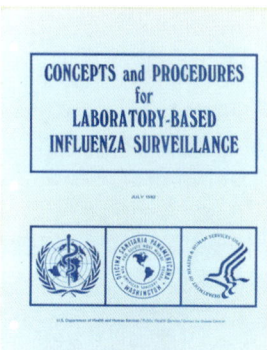
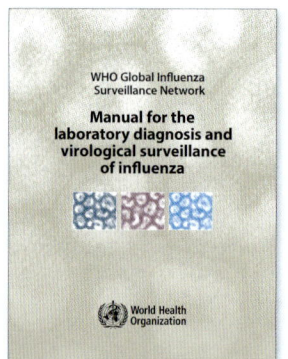

WHO efforts to nurture all of the vital collaborations needed to effectively coordinate and strengthen GISRS activities include the development and distribution of WHO guidelines, manuals, protocols and other documents to support national influenza surveillance activities. In addition, WHO will continue to offer regular evaluations of laboratory testing performance through its WHO external quality assessment programme, and to provide financial, technical and logistical assistance to NICs in the transporting of clinical specimens through the WHO Shipping Fund Project.

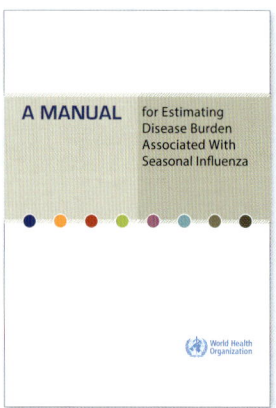
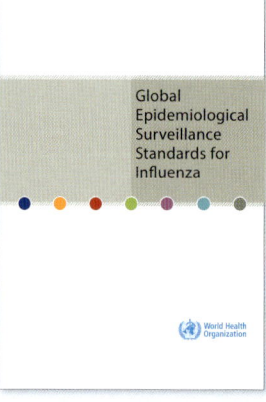

Making the case to national decision-makers for the importance of seasonal influenza vaccination will be dependent upon accurate estimates of the burden of influenza in countries, based upon sound epidemiological surveillance activities. The WHO *Manual for estimating disease burden associated with seasonal influenza* provides a standardized tool for influenza disease burden estimation in WHO Member States and is intended to be used in conjunction with the WHO *Global epidemiological surveillance standards for influenza*.

The WHO Shipping Fund Project provides financial and logistical support to NICs.

The safe and optimally timed transportation of influenza viruses between GISRS laboratories is one of the cornerstones of international collaboration against emerging and potentially dangerous influenza viruses. Because the infectivity of influenza viruses must be preserved for their subsequent analysis, their transportation must be done safely to avoid posing a threat to laboratory and transportation personnel. To address these and other associated challenges, the WHO Global Influenza Programme provides training on the safe handling of biological materials before, during and after transportation. In addition, the WHO Shipping Fund Project – a resource that was initially created to ensure the timely sharing of potentially pandemic avian influenza viruses – provides financial and logistical support to NICs to facilitate the sharing of seasonal influenza viruses.

Strict international regulations must be observed when shipping infectious substances both nationally and internationally. WHO provides training for NIC staff who upon successful completion of the course become formally qualified in the shipment of influenza viruses worldwide.

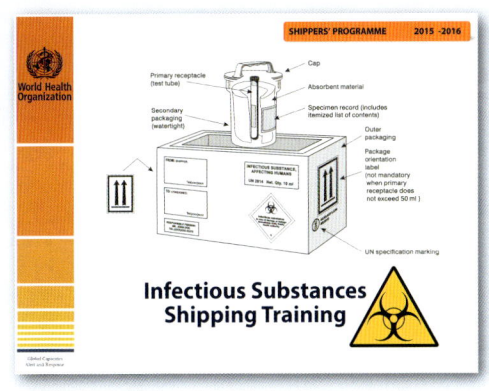

And it is not only within the human health sector that collaborations are nurtured and strengthened. In recent years, GISRS has intensified its collaboration with a range of networks and agencies conducting influenza surveillance in animals. Since 2005, OIE and FAO have collaborated through OFFLU. There is now intensive collaboration between GISRS and OFFLU at the interface of animal–human influenza, including through the joint investigation of zoonotic influenza outbreaks. In addition, during the biannual WHO vaccine composition meetings, OFFLU experts contribute essential information on influenza viruses causing outbreaks in wild and farmed animals. During these discussions, the group identifies potentially zoonotic variants of a range of animal influenza viruses. The identification of such viruses allows for an up-to-date collection of candidate vaccine viruses to be maintained for a wide range of pandemic preparedness and related purposes.

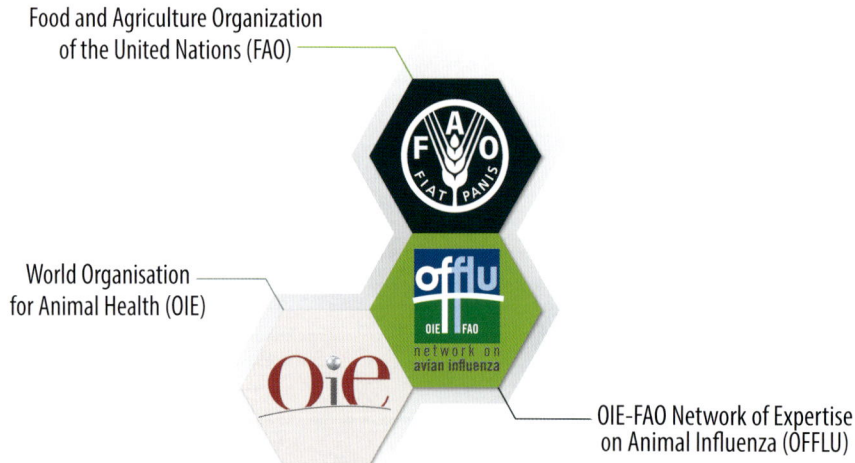

Another fundamental collaboration is the public–private partnership which exists between GISRS and vaccine manufactures, and which drives the production of both seasonal and pandemic influenza vaccines. Without this partnership, the production of such vaccines would simply not be possible. GISRS and the vaccine industry work together year round to ensure the timely production and availability of seasonal influenza vaccines. This involves close liaison in areas such as the selection and development of candidate vaccine viruses and regular teleconferences and other platforms for providing updates on vaccine production. During a pandemic, WHO will keep vaccine manufacturers updated on the virological and other data collected by GISRS laboratories, on the progression and severity of the pandemic, and on the availability of pandemic viruses for use in vaccine production. WHO will also receive information from vaccine manufacturers on the status of seasonal vaccine production and on the implications for both seasonal and pandemic vaccine supplies of switching to pandemic vaccine production at different times. WHO will then take this into account when deciding upon the optimal point at which to recommend the switch from seasonal to pandemic vaccine production.

GISRS is not the only network that focuses on the clinical, epidemiological, virological, pharmaceutical and public health aspects of influenza. Important partners here include but are not limited to the Asia-Pacific Alliance for the Control of Influenza (APACI); the Eastern Mediterranean Acute Respiratory Illness Surveillance Network (EMARIS); the Global Initiative on Sharing All Influenza Data (GISAID); the Global Approach to Biology in Response to Infectious Epidemics in Low-income Countries (GABRIEL); the Institut Pasteur International Network (RIIP); and the Global Health Network (GHN). Many of these networks work in close partnership with WHO and a number of institutes are part of both GISRS and other networks.

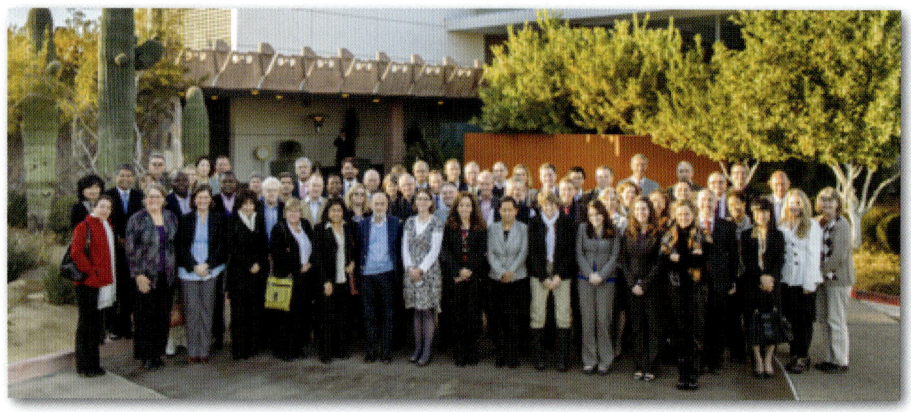

In January 2013, the International Influenza Networks Meeting in Scottsdale, Arizona, USA, brought together more than 30 networks focusing on various aspects of human and animal influenza.

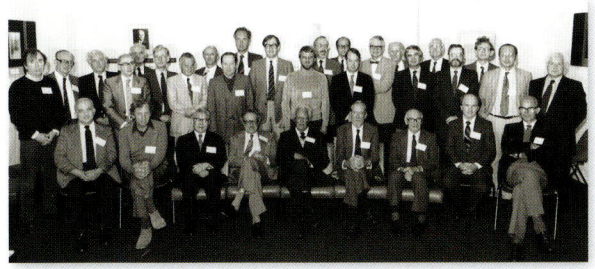

For the past 65 years, meetings have been an excellent and important way of bringing together people involved in influenza research and surveillance, in order to exchange the latest scientific information, develop ideas and plan joint projects. Many of the individuals in this picture are pioneers of influenza research.

If working together is the driving force of GISRS then face-to-face meetings – including the crucial biannual vaccine composition meetings – are its heartbeat. For almost seven decades, GISRS scientists, representatives of a wide range of partner organizations, agencies and other entities, and vaccine manufacturers have interacted at national, regional and international meetings, training workshops and courses. Such meetings also provide newcomers to the field with a valuable opportunity to meet colleagues from other countries and laboratories, exchange experiences and directly address problems and concerns. Many of the contacts established in such meetings have evolved into enduring professional collaborations.

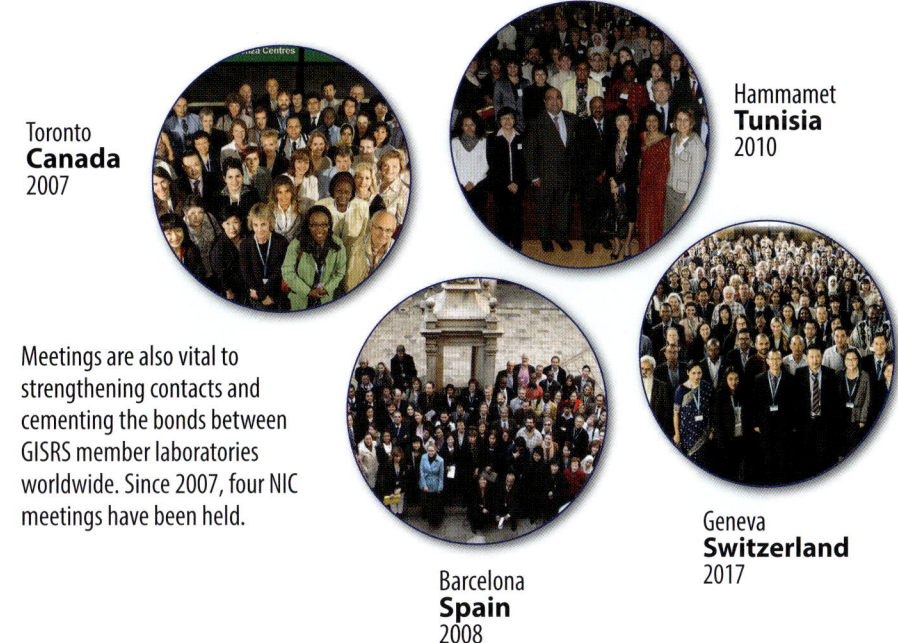

Toronto **Canada** 2007

Hammamet **Tunisia** 2010

Meetings are also vital to strengthening contacts and cementing the bonds between GISRS member laboratories worldwide. Since 2007, four NIC meetings have been held.

Barcelona **Spain** 2008

Geneva **Switzerland** 2017

New Technology Antigenic mapping
Close working Interconnected
Other emerging diseases Support developing countries Vaccine efficiency
Improved potential Respond rapidly Maintained role ONLINE
Software Real time Universal vaccine Next generation sequencing
Adaptable network Combat pandemics
User friendly
Bioinformatics Additional countries Shared findings
One Health Faster vaccines platforms
Larger network

Looking to the future

In 2017, almost exactly a century after the worst recorded pandemic in human history, GISRS reached its 65th anniversary of working at the forefront of the world's defences against influenza. Upon reaching such a milestone, it is natural to reflect upon such a long history and to commemorate some of the early pioneers whose vision made it all possible. However, it is also a time to look forward and to acknowledge that the work is not yet done.

Recent years have seen growing awareness by national governments and the international health community of the individual, social and economic burden of seasonal influenza. In addition, following the emergence of cases of highly pathogenic avian influenza in humans in 1997, long-standing concerns about the possibility of a human influenza pandemic have intensified, and were heightened again during the 2009 H1N1 pandemic. These and other factors have led to ever-increasing levels of demand by countries for WHO leadership and support in strengthening national, regional and international influenza surveillance, response and preparedness capabilities. In the face of such demands, GISRS will continue in its role as a highly responsive and adaptable global public health resource for the world. In order to achieve this aim, concerted efforts will continue to be made in:

- providing global leadership
- strengthening national capacities
- harnessing technology and furthering knowledge
- nurturing collaboration.

Providing global leadership

Because influenza viruses spread without regard to national borders, countermeasures have to be globally coordinated to have any chance of being effective. In addition, maximizing public health gains requires the optimum and equitable use of currently unevenly distributed critical capacities, such as vaccine production capacities. For as long as these and other realities remain, global leadership and coordination will be vital.

As the pre-eminent global public health entity for monitoring the constant threat of influenza, GISRS will continue to accumulate and share vital knowledge, and to guide and inform the activities and countermeasures to be taken – including the conducting of risk assessments and the development and updating of influenza vaccines. In parallel with this, GISRS will continue to advocate for the importance of this global public health priority, and to demonstrate to health policy-makers and donors the very significant health and economic benefits that would result from increased efforts in this area. In many countries, realizing these benefits will require the development of supportive national policies and sustainable capacity-building.

As demands for improvement continue to rise, national capacity-building will be the key to maintaining momentum and sustaining the gains already made. In countries currently lacking adequate influenza surveillance, decision-makers need to be alerted to the importance of influenza and other respiratory pathogens, suitably qualified laboratories need to be identified and sustainably supported, epidemiologists need to be trained, and communication channels need to be built. As part of this process, GISRS will continue to play a key role. For example, WHOCCs not only represent the pinnacle of technical leadership and world expertise on influenza, they have also invested millions of US dollars in providing world-class training to laboratory staff from around the world.

Strengthening national capacities

Following the re-emergence of human cases of H5N1 avian influenza in 2003 and the 2009 H1N1 pandemic, numerous WHO Member States increased their support for the GISRS laboratories that they generously host – thus taking an important step towards improved national influenza surveillance and response capacities. This is a welcome development but much more needs to be done if these gains are to be maintained and built upon, and the dangers of slipping back into complacency and under-funding are to be avoided. In many areas in the world the laboratory and epidemiological surveillance of seasonal influenza remains insufficient. In addition, detecting a single case of human infection with an unusual influenza virus – or even a small cluster of cases – would currently not occur promptly enough in many settings to allow for a timely response. These and many other gaps need to be filled if seasonal surveillance and global pandemic preparedness are to be taken to the next level.

GISRS will continue to act as a key mechanism for driving improvements in the context of broader international efforts such as the Joint External Evaluation process and IHR (2005) core capacity building in countries. As the platform through which countries can access the significant opportunities created by initiatives such as the landmark PIP Framework, GISRS is uniquely placed. Furthermore, using pandemic influenza as an example pathogen can be an invaluable entry point for strengthening national, regional and international all-hazards preparedness, while simultaneously strengthening GISRS. As NICs in many countries are often the front-line institution for responding to other highly dangerous pathogens such as the MERS coronavirus and Ebola virus, such efforts will inevitably strengthen overall national – and thus global – health security.

Harnessing technology and furthering scientific understanding

The spirit and enthusiasm shown by those early scientists who first succeeded in demonstrating beyond doubt the viral nature of influenza and isolating the causative viruses have continued unabated throughout the 65-year history of GISRS and will continue to do so. Creative and groundbreaking individuals, captivated by the fascinating biology and epidemiology of influenza viruses, will continue to drive forward technological developments – frequently at the cutting edge of scientific understanding. Without the advances made throughout its history, many of the public health achievements of GISRS would not have been possible. Similarly, without the willingness by GISRS to adopt and be open to exciting new technologies and advances in knowledge, there will be no revolutionary breakthroughs in influenza surveillance, prevention and control.

For example, the advent of routine next-generation sequencing brings with it the promise of a fundamental paradigm shift in GISRS activities. In the future, it may be possible to first sequence large numbers of influenza virus genomes directly from clinical samples and to use the data generated to select viruses for detailed antigenic analysis. At the same time, approaches such as synthetic genomics; systems genetics, biology and immunology; and mathematical modelling are all capable of generating enormous volumes of highly complex and diverse data that can be applied to influenza prevention and control. Delivering on the promises of the future and harnessing the currently theoretical benefits of these and other potentially revolutionary advances will depend upon the continuing efforts of dedicated GISRS laboratories worldwide and on the close collaboration and engagement of GISRS with scientists working in many different disciplines.

Microarray technology will increasingly be used for the detection and identification of viral nucleic acids in a technique called Advanced Molecular Detection. Using this technique, the detailed genetic characteristics of individual influenza viruses can be obtained within hours.

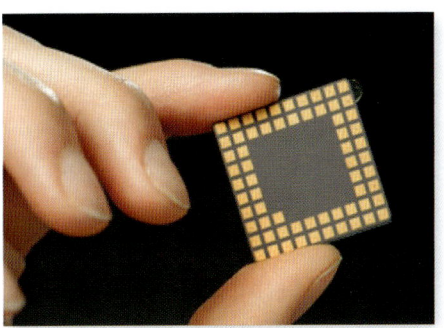

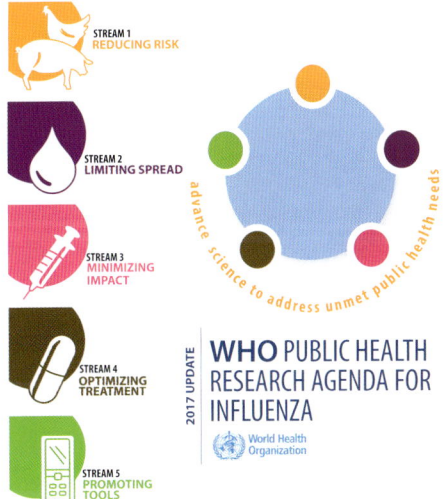

For as long as influenza continues to be a major public health threat, GISRS will also continue to play its part in driving research to further knowledge. The WHO Public Health Research Agenda for Influenza is organized around a framework of five research streams with particular relevance to the public health aspects of influenza.

Nurturing vital collaborations

Lying at the heart of global influenza surveillance and control efforts, GISRS will continue to nurture and channel the enthusiasm and collective spirit of all its member entities and partners. Minimizing the public health impact and socioeconomic burdens of influenza and ensuring preparedness for the next influenza pandemic will continue to rely upon the support of national governments, and on the interaction as equal partners of NICs, WHOCCs, WHO ERLs and WHO H5 Reference Laboratories worldwide. In addition, countless scientists, doctors, nurses, veterinarians and technicians working in research and epidemiological institutes and in the animal influenza sector have already demonstrated their willingness to work together for a common cause. And to these we must add the donors, vaccine manufacturers and others in the private sector, without whose support and collaboration very little would be possible. As part of nurturing these and other vital collaborations, regional and global meetings of GISRS and its partners will continue to provide invaluable opportunities to disseminate information and ideas, and to realize the incalculable benefits of face-to-face contact.

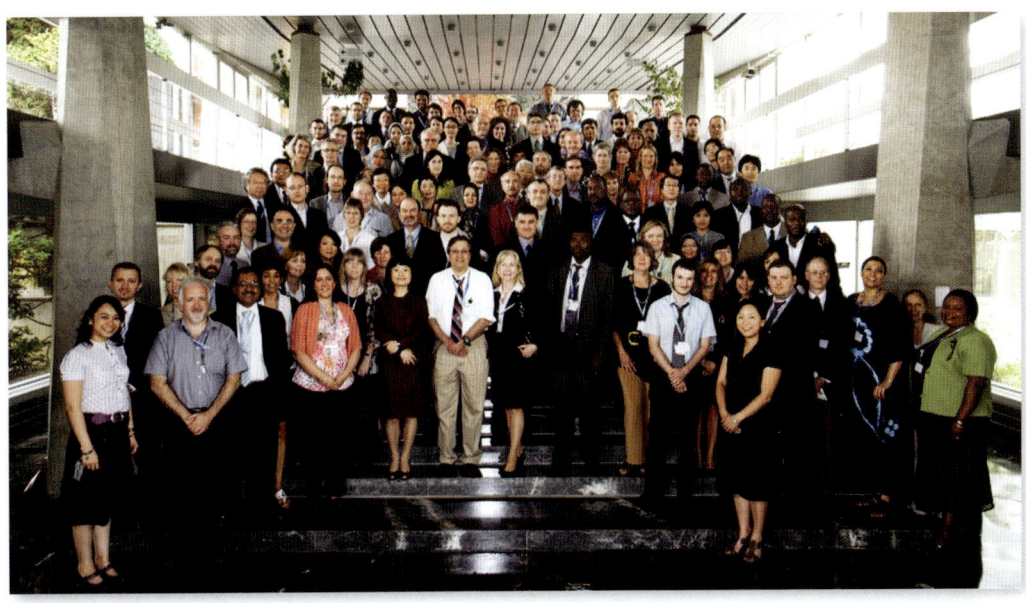

Since 2010 WHO has held a series of informal consultations on improving influenza vaccine virus selection. These meetings have epitomized the commitment of GISRS to strategically provide its support in the key areas of providing global leadership, promoting national capacity-building, harnessing new technologies and nurturing vital collaborations. Such events have provided valuable opportunities for in-depth discussions of developments in national influenza surveillance and response activities, of exciting developments in laboratory and vaccine-production technologies, and of the latest advances made in related fields such as the mathematical modelling of viral evolution. The meetings bring together a highly diverse range of representatives from regulatory authorities, the vaccine industry, the animal influenza surveillance sector, academia and other stakeholders.

The GISRS Journey

Thirty years after the 1918 Spanish flu pandemic, the deadliest such pandemic in recorded history and one of the worst natural disasters ever to confront the human race, the vision of mounting a global effort against influenza began to take shape. Shortly afterwards, in 1952, GISRS was established, and since then it has proven to be a unique and enduring global health collaboration. To this day, almost seven decades later, GISRS remains an exemplar of international health cooperation without parallel.

Built on the collaborative efforts of generations of dedicated scientists and public health officials, GISRS has grown from its European-centred beginnings to become a truly global health and health security resource for the whole world. Today, more than 150 institutions in well over a hundred countries provide the vital information and viruses needed to respond year round to the recurring epidemics of seasonal influenza and to maintain the constant vigilance that is so crucial if the world is to be given any warning of the onset of the next pandemic.

In a world that, like the influenza virus itself, is constantly evolving and changing such vigilance is indeed crucial. As demographic, economic and environmental realities bring increasing numbers of people into ever closer proximity to the animal virus reservoir, and as the sheer scale and ease of international travel continue to grow, so too the opportunities for the next human-adapted animal virus to emerge and spread. History and science tell us that this spread is likely to be very rapid and to carry within it the potential to bring untold human suffering and economic devastation in its wake. When the window of opportunity for protecting millions is likely to be narrow, the need for the constant monitoring, continual risk evaluation and rapid response that only GISRS can provide could not be clearer.

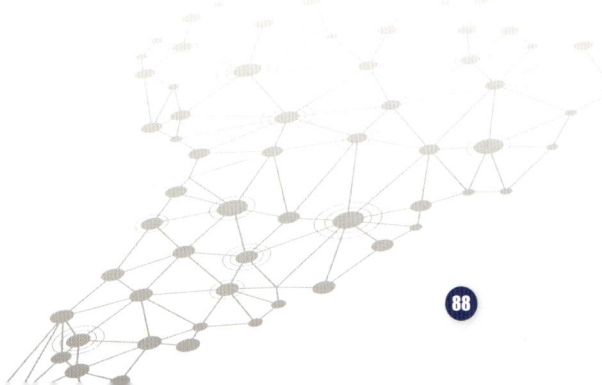

In order to meet the many challenges it will undoubtedly face in the coming years and decades, GISRS, under the coordination of WHO, will continue to advocate for and support national, regional and global efforts to strengthen seasonal and pandemic influenza surveillance and response capabilities. GISRS will also continue to drive and harness new scientific and technological advances that have the potential to dramatically enhance our understanding of virus evolution and spread, and to revolutionize influenza vaccine development and production. And above all else, the current guardians of GISRS will work to nurture new and existing partnerships, to expand collaboration and to preserve that sense of a shared endeavour for the common good that has been its driving force from the very beginning.

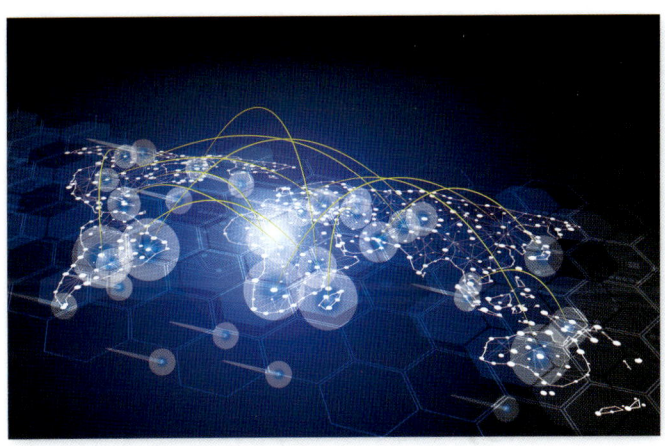